Genetically engineered food, free radicals, and other apocalyptic scenarios are explored and practical solutions offered in this uniquely informative new herbal. Here is an herb book that not only provides the kind of practical information one has come to expect from a good herbal, but additionally provides a sweeping overview of herbal medicine and its role in the current environmental and health crisis. Madonna Sophia Compton has written an intelligent treatise on the modern day health crisis and explains in clear terms how by using simple earth remedies we participate in restoring health and balance for the planet and ourselves. —ROSEMARY GLADSTAR, AUTHOR OF "HERBAL HEALING FOR WOMEN"

Dr. Christopher is pure in the sense of Hippocrates: that is, the body heals itself if given the right environment. —INTERVIEW WITH DR. CHRISTOPHER'S SON DAVID IN "HERBAL GOLD"

If the germs—our modern demons—are mutating and getting stronger, we need to compensate by creating an even healthier immune system. —MADONNA SOPHIA COMPTON

An Herbal for the New Millennium

Herbal Gold contains the latest research to help you make healthy resolutions for the coming millennium. With the expert help of herbalist and holistic healing expert Madonna Sophia Compton, you can learn to use the right herbs in the right combinations to:

- boost your immune system
- increase longevity
- cure nutritional deficiencies
- treat illnesses and injuries
- reduce stress
- improve your spirit
- foster resilience in all areas of your life

Let *Herbal Gold* be your guide on the road to a healthier lifestyle and a renewal of mental and physical power.

About the Author

Madonna Sophia Compton has been active in the alternative health movement for twenty-five years. She facilitates women's menopause and midlife groups in the Bay Area and is a resident herbalist at the Sonoma Holistic Center, where she does consultations. She spent years growing and studying the magic of herbs on a farm in the Missouri Ozarks before moving to California eleven years ago. She is a member of the Herb Research Foundation and teaches at the Graduate School for Holistic Studies at John F. Kennedy University in Orinda, California, where she received her masters degree. Her primary orientation in terms of herbal philosophy is the Dr. Christopher School for Natural Healing. In 1997, she was Vice President of Product Research for a major herb company and then went on to start her own organic herb store with bulk herbs, teas, spices, and aromatherapy oils. For information about herb walks and classes, write The Herb Farm, 7110 Hwy. 29, Kelseyville, CA 95451.

To Write to the Author

If you wish to contact the author or would like more information about this book, please write to the author in care of Llewellyn Worldwide and we will forward your request. Both the author and publisher appreciate hearing from you and learning of your enjoyment of this book and how it has helped you. Llewellyn Worldwide cannot guarantee that every letter written to the author can be answered, but all will be forwarded. Please write to:

Madonna Sophia Compton
℅ Llewellyn Worldwide
P.O. Box 64383, Dept. K172-4
St. Paul, MN 55164-0383, U.S.A.

Please enclose a self-addressed stamped envelope for reply, or $1.00 to cover costs. If outside U.S.A., enclose international postal reply coupon.

HEALING ALTERNATIVES

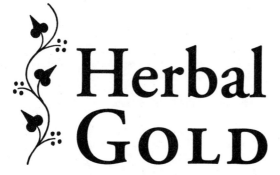

Herbal GOLD

The complete guide to the use,
lore and application of over 90
essential medicinal herbs

MADONNA SOPHIA COMPTON

2000
Llewellyn Publications
St. Paul, Minnesota 55164-0383, U.S.A.

First Edition
First Printing, 2000

Book design and editing by Rebecca Zins
Cover design by Anne Marie Garrison

Permission to quote from the following sources is gratefully acknowledged: *Herbal Pathfinders* ©1983 by Robert Conrow and Arlene Hecksel; David Christopher of Christopher Enterprises; Rosemary Gladstar.

Library of Congress Cataloging-in-Publication Data
Compton, Madonna, 1947-
   Herbal gold: healing alternatives: the complete guide to the use, lore, and application of over 90 essential medicinal herbs / Madonna Sophia Compton.—1st ed.
      p.   cm.
   ISBN 1-56718-172-4
   1. Herbs—Therapeutic use.   2. Materia medica, Vegetable.   I. Title.
RM666.H33 C676 2000
615'.321—dc21
                                                                  99-054457

Llewellyn Publications
A Division of Llewellyn Worldwide, Ltd.
P.O. Box 64383, Dept. K172-4
St. Paul, MN 55164-0383, U.S.A.
www.llewellyn.com

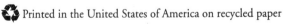 Printed in the United States of America on recycled paper

Other Books by
Madonna Sophia Compton

Women at the Change: The Intelligent Woman's
Guide to Menopause
(Llewellyn, 1997)

Archetypes on the Tree of Life
(Llewellyn, 1995)

*T*his book is dedicated
to my mother,
my greatest inspiration
for a hopeful future.

Contents

Part II

Part III

Preface

Growing, harvesting, eating, and studying herbs has been a favorite pastime of mine ever since I was a young mother almost thirty years ago. Living in a farm in the rural Missouri Ozarks, we had little resources available except what we grew, stored, and dried ourselves. Perhaps once a month we would make the eighty-mile trip to town for supplies. But we certainly could not get in the car and go out for a quick loaf of bread or some aspirin! And we would only go in for a doctor's visit on rare occasions (usually dire emergencies), preferring to investigate alternative models of holistic healing ourselves.

Today I often see young couples taking their babies to the doctor (usually for antibiotics prescriptions) every few weeks or months. This is an alarming trend and reflects, as we will be discussing, a growing tendency toward decreased immune function. One thing I grew to be deeply grateful for during my farm years was the power of herbal home-cures. After I moved back to the city and started a teaching and writing career, I began researching herbs and other holistic models in a more academically rigorous fashion, and my fascination with both the mystery and the science of healing plants continued to grow.

I have watched the herbal industry go through many changes over the past three decades, from the discovery of the great teachers of the early nineteenth century by the counterculture in the '60s—greats like Jethro Kloss and John Christopher—to the more modern applications of studying the effects of herbal medicines under strict laboratory conditions. Throughout, there has grown a steady interest on the part of the general public in what these magical plants are up to. How do they exert their healing power in some people and not in others? How do they have such a large range of therapeutic action? How can they be used to replace more harmful, synthetic drugs and their uncomfortable side effects?

Many questions remain to be answered, but there are some wonderful teachers and many resources upon which one may begin to journey with the healing foods God has placed on this planet. I hope this book serves as a useful addition to the growing body of literature on how to interact with the herbal kingdom, for in my opinion, there is very little on this earth that is as valuable as herbal gold.

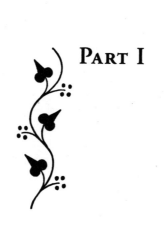

PART I

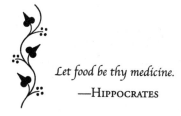

Let food be thy medicine.
   —Hippocrates

1

The Emergence of Herbal Gold

We are in the presence of a renaissance, or paradigm shift, in many disciplines as we enter the new millennium. Herbal medicine is no exception. Although viewed with scorn and skepticism by American science and medicine for the past 100 years, the renewed interest in what Mother Nature has to offer, ironically, is coming principally from these very disciplines. There has been an enormous influx in scientific investigation into the use of plant medicines the past two decades.

Herbalism, an arcane tradition once shrouded in mystery and understood only by a select few, is now open to research and technological development. This has advantages, but it also has a downside. Although organic formulations from nature are now being made available to huge numbers of people, there is the risk that, by taking specific components of a herb isolated from the rest of the plant, we encounter the possibility of increased toxicity, or unwanted side effects, which can happen because a herb is not administered holistically. (More about this later.) In the past, there has not been a clear boundary between plants, food, herbs, and plant medicines. All are derived from nature and are used to keep the body functioning at optimum health. We need to remember the injunction of Hippocrates if we want to reclaim our healthy birthright, rather than think we can "improve" on nature.

Nonetheless, there are benefits to the growing interest in doing scientific studies on traditional herbs and incorporating this knowledge into modern pharmacology. Two decades ago, almost none of the major pharmaceutical companies had plant research programs; by the mid-1990s, pharmaceuticals derived from plants were a $10 billion business in the United States, primarily because of the increased public awareness and demand for medicinal products that were plant-derived.[1] In addition, the age of preventive medicine is now upon us and, as time goes on, more phytonutrients are being discovered in plants that not only treat but help prevent disease when incorporated into a daily diet. Many noted physicians and scientists are now seeing a link between the routine use of natural supplements (combined with good dietary habits) and the lower incidence of degenerative diseases.

Between 1996 and 1999, I maintained a website where I had the opportunity to act as a consultant for people who had questions about herbs and minerals or who needed information about resources for menopause and midlife health. Both of these forums were productive avenues, not only for me to offer whatever service I could, but also to discern the prevalent problems and symptoms plaguing modern civilized society. I became so concerned about the nature of some of these major health and environmental concerns that I decided to write this book, attempting to address how a holistic approach, using herbs and whole food supplements, can help realign balance and restore health and vitality in our otherwise very sick, unbalanced, and polluted world. I feel very strongly that the bounty given to us by Mother Nature holds the key to correcting many of these ills, and in this herbal I have attempted to address not only the traditional uses and folklore of herbs—a fascination of mine for many years—but also the more recent scientific discoveries about specific herbal actions and properties. Nature's pharmacy, in my opinion, has much more to offer in maintaining optimum health than does a synthetic drug design. Many times I see clients who complain of the side effects of these "miracle drugs," e.g., joint pain from cholesterol-lowering drugs, high blood pressure from a number of medications, weight gain from anti-depressants. As I explored in my last book, *Women at the Change,* the side effects from hormone replacement therapy are so numerous, the list would not fit onto just one page! These are the reasons we need to turn to natural methods of healing. Today, we are rediscovering the great value of herbal gold and the power it has to restore good health.

In the course of working with people in my personal and on-line consulting, I have discovered that there are a number of frequently asked questions. I have included them here. For a fuller examination of some of these issues, see the chapters that follow.

Frequently Asked Questions About Herbs

What are phytonutrients?

Phytonutrients simply refer to the nutrient-dense elements in plants ("phyto") that are responsible for plants' healing properties. Phytotherapy is the term used to describe the practice of herbal medicine in European countries. Phytotherapy is the science of using plants for medicine. It has become somewhat fashionable to use these terms to describe the aspects of plant-foods that are both healing and preventative, as the United States catches up with the other 80 percent of the world that uses herbs regularly.

Should I take herbs all the time or only when I am sick?

A good rule is to use herbs in moderation, not only to feel better but also to maintain optimum health. Some phytonutrients and herbs can be used on a daily basis as a preventive measure against disease. In treating specific illnesses, targeted herbs should be administered for short periods of time in stronger doses.

How often should I take herbs?

A good suggestion is to start with one or two capsules twice a day for herbs that are whole-food based, that is, that are used in place of synthetic vitamins. Then as you build up to it, or see effective results, the dosage may be increased to up to two capsules, three times a day. In treating particular disorders, it is generally advisable to follow directions in an herbal guide for teas, extracts, and so on, or directions printed on the bottle, if taken in capsule form. These herbs should always be taken with a large glass of water.

Can I take more than one herbal product at a time?

Yes, it is fine to take herbs singly or in combination. However, some herbs should not be combined (e.g., a stimulant and a sedative, or two herbs that both have a strong effect on blood sugar or the heart, e.g., ma-huang and ginseng). I have discussed this problem more in chapter 4. In addition, it is best not to use herbs consistently. That is, it is most beneficial to take a break from herbs. Most herbalists use the 1:7 rule. Normally taking one day off a week is suggested, even when treating symptoms. In this way, the body is more able to effectively use herbs.

How long does it take to see the effects of herbs?

Every individual is different. Results depend on a variety of factors, including how often and with what consistency herbs are taken. Many see results almost immediately: they feel more alive, have better focus, more energy, and so on. If you have a health problem, you should expect to take herbs over an extended period of time before seeing significant improvement. In using herbs as supplements to protect your overall health, it is best to rotate the kind of herb one is using for optimum benefit. For example, you may want to take some liver-detoxing herbs for a few weeks, then some herbs that cleanse the kidney, then some that purify and build the blood, and so on. Some herbs are whole-food based and, like supplements, can be used with greater regularity. Garlic, ginkgo, and Siberian ginseng are examples of herbs that can be used more frequently.

Are there side effects when taking these herbs?

Herbs are a natural food designed by Mother Nature to work with the body in promoting health and vitality. However, when ingested into a toxic body loaded with chemical pollutants that have been ingested over a long period of time, there may be some detox reactions. These may include diarrhea, skin eruptions, headache, or congestion. The rule of thumb, however, if this is occurring, is to cut back on the dosage rather than quit. If you continue to have serious side effects from a particular herb, consult your health-care practitioner.

If I have more than one physical symptom, should I treat them separately or together?

Most herbalists believe it is not productive to take too many herbs at one time, although some herbs complement one another quite well. It is best, in this regard, to have the advice of a holistic practitioner. A general rule recommended by one great herbalist, Dr. John Christopher, is that one "cleanse and nourish" with specific herbs; then look to herbs and phytonutrients as a food to build the body back to health.[2] Once again, contraindications should be observed; that is, some herbs are inadvisable to take together.

Can I take herbs with prescribed medicines?

Herbs can sometimes be taken with prescribed medication. However, it is advisable to seek expert advice, ideally a practitioner who understands the benefits of herbs and their actions as well as the type of medication prescribed. Medications should be cut in half if they are being used to treat the same symptoms as the herb (for example, for weight loss or for depression). Many people find that they can discontinue their medications altogether eventually.

Are there any contraindications in using herbs?

There can be, especially if the herb is standardized. (Standardization uses chemicals to isolate the active ingredients from the other constituents that make up an herb.) If using the whole herb, as in a tea, for example, most herbs are very safe. Always check with your holistic practitioner if you are uncertain, especially if you are on prescribed medications.

Is it advisable to give herbs to children?

Yes, with the exception of herbs like ma-huang, which have a strong stimulating effect, or some of the sedative or antidepressant herbs, it is safe to give children herbs in less amounts, and they generally experience very good results. The general rule is half an adult dose for teens and older children, and a quarter dose or less for younger children.

Do I need to change my diet when I take herbs?

Ideally, it is advisable to avoid alcohol, smoking, and the ever-available junk foods, especially prepackaged or laced with a lot of chemical preservatives, to benefit the most from taking herbs and phytonutrients. This is particularly true of one suffers from ADD (attention deficit disorder) or chronic immune system deficiency diseases. Any herbal program works best when combined with a natural foods diet.

What are the main actions of herbs?

Principally they are cleansing, building, and nourishing. Some herbs help cleanse and purify the body, especially the liver and bloodstream. Herbal builders regulate and tone the glands to function in the best condition. Nourishing herbs are exceptionally high in vitamins and minerals and other nutrients that are essential to good health. In addition, herbs can sedate or stimulate. This is only a brief overview.

At the beginning of each herb described in the herbal section of this book, there is a section called "Therapeutic Profile" that lists the specific action of the herb. One can then check the glossary of herbal actions for a description of that particular action.

What is the difference between taking a herb and a drug?

Herbs are natural remedies that work with the body to heal disease and maintain good health. They generally do not have the serious side effects that are common to most of the prescribed drugs available today. However, many drugs are synthesized from herbs. Aspirin, for instance, is a chemical imitation of salicin from white willow bark. Digitalis is the active principle of foxglove. Natural substances, however, cannot be patented. In isolating and frequently changing the chemical composition of herbal constituents, the functions of their active chemicals are often changed or altered. This is necessary in order for the pharmaceutical companies to manufacture and prescribe drugs, so they can make a good deal of money in the process.

With very few exceptions, herbs are much safer and frequently are more effective than drugs, especially when taken over a long period of time.

What are the principal benefits from taking herbs as opposed to drugs or synthetic vitamins?

Herbs produce a feeling of natural wellness and vital energy. One often experiences the ability to rebound from stressful situations easily. Many report an increased mental alertness or expanded awareness. There is much evidence that the immune system is made stronger and is more effective in protecting one from disease. Often, people are able to experience a nutritional way to keep extra pounds off. The results are limitless. Drugs generally treat symptoms and not the underlying cause of disease and, in addition, often cause more serious problems in the long run.

Some herbs are standardized, and approach a synthesized version of medicine that have effects similar to drug actions; nonetheless, they are made from natural sources and their chemical composition has not been altered, as in the case with most drugs. More on the standardization debate follows in later chapters.

One of the most important reasons why it is important to supplement one's diet with herbs and mineral-rich foods is for protection, detoxification, and the vital nourishment lacking because of the very polluted state of the world right now. It is my belief that modern doctors have made great strides in human health care, particularly in providing critical care, and their work is to be commended. However, thanks to some of the repercussions of the pharmaceutical industry and most doctors' reliance upon it, we are dying long, painful, expensive deaths and we are plagued with degenerative diseases half of our lives.

Notes

1. Michael Weiner and Janet Weiner, *Herbs That Heal* (Mill Valley, CA: Quantum Books, 1994), p. 46.
2. Dr. John Christopher. See his "mucousless diet" theory, available from Christopher Publications, and his classic text, an herbal therapy book, *School of Natural Healing* (Springville, Utah: Christopher Publications, 1976).

*We are waiting for the millennium, but before that time comes,
we may go through a great deal of hard times and tribulation.
Some of us will be prepared to survive the holocaust or
natural disasters that may occur, and others will be
as unprepared as a featherless turkey in a snowstorm.*

—DR. JOHN CHRISTOPHER

2

Apocalyptic Scenarios and What You Can Do About Them

*A*nyone who picks up this book has probably already made a decision. It may be a decision to change personal eating habits based on what we now know about the poisons in our food chain, or it may be a more global commitment to affect changes that may, in fact, tip the scales in favor of saving our planet from extinction. At any rate, congratulations on your decision: you have inquired about options. You have opened the door to explore alternatives. You have inquired about herbal opportunities that can offer health, balance, and creative solutions in a world that, as we move into the twenty-first century, can often seem to hold very little promise.

The fact is, there are more degenerative diseases today than ever before: cancer, heart disease, and arthritis abound, as well as numerous allergic reactions, a variety of immune system deficiencies, severe PMS symptoms that were almost unheard of a generation or two ago, viruses that mutate faster than we can keep up with, and hyperactivity and attention deficit disorders in our children.

We have to honestly ask ourselves why we, and not earlier generations who ate nutrient-rich foods often grown on their own farms, suffer these disorders in such huge numbers. Could it be related to the fact that we are ingesting more toxins from our food and environment than ever before in human history?

Most of us know that planetary pollution has reached startling and dangerous proportions in the past fifty years, due to the overuse of pesticides and herbicides; our dependence on overirrigation; the severe depletion of our topsoil; and the toxic wastes dumped into our rivers, oceans, and even the air we breathe. From New York City to the deepest recesses of the Amazon jungle, no part of our planet has remained untouched by the vast and ugly reach of our "pollution monsters." This has, of course, far-reaching consequences for the planet and immediate consequences for ourselves, our families, and the next generation.

What is very frightening to many scientists is not only the use of single toxic pesticides on our foods but now the synergistic effect of numerous ones combined, which can increase the harmful, degenerative, disease-causing effects of these chemicals exponentially. A study released to the Associated Press indicated pesticides that by themselves had been linked to various cancers are 1,000 times more potent when combined. The Environmental Protection Agency called the results of this study "astonishing."[1] As if that were not enough, after food is harvested, hundreds of chemical additives and preservatives are added to them, many of which have never even had FDA approval. They preserve food on its long journey from the farm to the supermarket, keep it looking pretty, add artificial flavors when the natural ones fade away, improve texture, and make it unappealing to bugs. The list of reasons for the use of food additives is endless, but the bottom line is always the same: unnatural foods tamper with health unnaturally.

In addition to these problems—with which many of us are already familiar—there are a number of serious hazards that are just beginning to surface in the media, but which have been a concern to many people working in the area of holistic health or environmental awareness for quite some time. And unfortunately they have consequences that could border on the apocalyptic. When one begins to examine the research, it becomes very apparent that unless these challenges are faced and creative solutions begin to unfold soon, the next century may look very grim indeed. I am going to discuss these problems briefly, then move on to something a lot more promising: this book is about positive approaches to health using the gifts of the herbal kingdom. My hope is that, in the process of becoming informed consumers, we can be instrumental in helping to shift awareness to an ecological consciousness that will no longer tolerate the blatant abuses to the earth and its creatures that we have in the past. And, of course, we can each try to personally include enough of the protective nutrients discussed in this book to help shield ourselves from the consequences of these potential disasters. More about that later.

The main crises I see looming on the horizon demanding our immediate attention are:

- Hormone disrupters
- Mad cow and related diseases
- Radiation and toxic waste
- Genetically engineered foods
- Overuse of antibiotics and emerging diseases, including potential biological warfare
- The depletion of our topsoil (This will be discussed in the next chapter.)

Let's take them one at a time.

Hormone Disruptors

Although there are many carcinogens that have been identified in numerous pesticides, herbicides, and other chemicals in our environment, there are a particular class of them that have become known as hormone disrupters, or xenoestrogens, that are particularly frightening. I discussed this briefly in my book *Women at the Change*, and only became aware of the issue's magnitude through my correspondence with Dr. John Lee when consulting with him for that book.[2] However, the earliest effects of this problem can be traced back for at least twenty years. Unfortunately, it is only when the tip of the iceberg emerges that we begin to sense the potential apocalyptic consequences of what we have been doing to the planet and to ourselves.

The first estrogen mimic, diethylstilbestrol (DES), affected more than 10 million people. Many women faced miscarriages, vaginal and cervical cancers, and other gynecological problems, and many men developed genital abnormalities and low sperm counts because their mothers took DES while pregnant. By the time the FDA issued warnings about it, it was much too late. We now know that there are equally dangerous estrogen mimics, or xenoestrogens, in our environment that are wreaking havoc not only with the human population but with an unknown number of other species as well.

The hormone disrupters that most closely resemble the estrogen molecule are primarily found in PCBs and plastics. This means that when ingested—and xenoestrogens from both PCBs and plastics do leak into foods—the body believes that these are really hormones, and the hormone receptor (sometimes referred to as the "lock") is opened by the hormone mimic (the "key"). Up until this generation, these locks and keys have been strictly bound together in the natural way they have always occurred together in the body.

Once activated, hormones can then cause the genes to act in a certain way. Studies have uncovered numerous instances wherein women who had eaten PCB-contaminated fish had children who suffered from low birth weight and neurological impairment,[3] which are some of the consequences of altering the body's normal hormonal activity. The implications of this alteration undermine the reproductive health of potentially millions of people, as well as many kinds of animals living today. Perhaps most distressing is how it may affect our innocent children for generations.

Have you ever wondered why the sperm count is declining? Accounts range from 25 to 40 percent over the past twenty years.[4] Every now and then the media will run a short story on it, only to quickly brush it under the table. However, according to Dr. Robert Kavlock, who directs the reproductive toxicology division of the EPA, the causes and effects of hormone disruption are "the number one environmental issue in toxicology right now."[5]

Most of us have heard of the tragic stories of the damage done to wildlife: sterility or reproductive failure in some species, abnormally small penises or grotesque deformities in others. Bald eagles, alligators, frogs, and mink are only a few of the species now being investigated. Many appear destined for extinction. Theo Colborn examines the evidence that has accumulated for both humans and wildlife in her landmark book *Our Stolen Future.*[6] She and her colleagues reviewed over 5,000 studies and consulted with hundreds of scientists around the world. Together, the literature documents an alarming and rapidly growing array of effects from these endocrine disrupters, including thyroid disorders, birth deformities, reduced immune response, neurological and behavioral changes, disrupted sexual development, and infertility. Some wildlife species have been reported to have deformed genitalia, aberrant mating behavior, and sterility.

It is quite possible that the mysterious hormone problems facing many more women today than in previous generations, from early menstruation and recurrent PMS to infertility and severe menopause, are linked to these environmental hormone disrupters. Studies have indicated that women working on pesticide-laden farms were twenty times more likely to be infertile as other women.[7] One study of 17,000 girls revealed the alarming data that up to 48 percent of them were developing breasts and/or pubic hair by age eight, and some as early as age four.[8] In Texas, the presence of one xenoestrogen, bisphenol-A, was found to be exceptionally high in the soil and linked to the region's high incidence of neural birth defects. Studies now reveal that the unborn may, in fact, be at very high risk.[9] Scientists are so concerned about this problem that a number of conferences have been held around the world to discuss the latest findings and possible consequences. At one in northern California a few years ago, according to my interview with Dr. John Lee, one scientist ventured to suggest that the last male to father a child in the United States may have already been born.[10]

Signs of hormone dysfunction may not have been noticed too overtly by this generation, but they will certainly show up in the next one if consciousness is not raised about this issue. Also, we may not have noticed the subtle impacts of endocrine disruption already because some of the effects—neurological and intelligence response, reproductive tract abnormalities, deficient immune response, improper hormonal balance, infertility, and cancer—have all been attributed to alternate factors. However, the xenoestrogen link is certainly one to be aware of. The alarming rise in breast cancer is a case in point.

Studies now indicate that the xenoestrogenic link may be a preventable cause of breast cancer.[11] In some places, when a xenoestrogenic pesticide is banned, breast cancer rates appear to drop dramatically, indicating that our increased use of pesticide-laden foods the past twenty years is a known source of cancer and other female disorders.[12] Numerous studies now are seeing clear evidence that breast fat serum lipids of women with breast cancer contain significantly elevated levels of these environmental carcinogens.[13] Yet these stories never seem to make the 6 o'clock news.

Although you may not be reading about it in the paper, tests are being conducted all over the world revealing the link between hormone disrupters and numerous anomalies and abnormalities. They are much too numerous to document in detail here. In some cases, the ingestion of these chemicals during pregnancy is critical to the health of the fetus. For example, pregnant rats fed one meal per day containing a small percentage of dioxin will produce offspring with smaller sex organs, a 75 percent reduction in sperm counts, and feminized sexual behavior.[14]

And although the media appears to be uncomfortably quiet about the potentially grave consequences of this issue, the government has designated the EPA to develop testing strategies for hormone disrupters and submit a report to Congress by the end of the year 2000. A special committee has been formed to examine this problem in depth, called the Endocrine Disrupter Screening and Testing Advisory Committee, with members from the Departments of Agriculture, Defense, Energy, and the Interior, as well as the EPA, the FDA, the National Cancer Institute, the National Science Foundation, and numerous environmental groups.[15] They compose a pretty diverse group of people working together to do a complete review of this rapidly growing tragic phenomenon.

As usual, the U.S. government will probably "study" the problem indefinitely before taking concrete action, such as the sensible banning of certain chemical agents and industrial byproducts, and an examination of alternatives to our overuse of plastics. However, in some countries, such as Denmark and Switzerland, some chemical agents that are clearly xenoestrogenic have already been banned or restrictions have been placed on their use. Canada has issued an informational brochure called "Reducing your Risk," available from the Canadian Wildlife Association.

What can you do to reduce your risk of exposure to these dangerous chemicals so that you can protect yourself and the future health of your children?

- Cut down on meat and dairy fats, since the concentration of many xenoestrogens tends to be in animal fat. Or else try and make sure these products come from organic sources. Likewise, avoid fish that have a high fat content unless you are sure that it comes from unpolluted sources.

- Do not use anything plastic (even though it may be advertised as heat-resistant) in a microwave. Always use ceramic or glass, and do not use Styrofoam at all. Try not to use plastic bottles and tops for children, particularly if they chew on them.

- Discourage pesticides in your local parks and schoolyards. Be especially aware of the pollutants from highly industrial areas— many of these are xenoestrogens. The ones presently in the spotlight are the dioxins, flurans, and PCBs. Inquire about ones used often in farming areas that are dangerous: atrazine, chlordane, chlordecone, DDT, DDE, and lindane.

- Don't use detergents, cosmetics, or shampoos with alkylphenol ethoxylates (APEs), nonoxynols, octoxynols, or lindane. Best yet, try to get these products organically.

- Research the herbs and phytonutrients in this book. There are many studies that now demonstrate the effectiveness of some of these God-given medicinal and nutrient-dense plants in protecting one from the possible effects of toxicity. Endocrine disrupters, like other chemical agents, tear down the immune response. Many nutrients can greatly aid in restoring hormonal balance and rebuilding the immune system, even when certain symptoms are already evident. Scan the charts and look at the studies.

The sad fact is that these chemicals have penetrated to the ends of the earth. The chemical evidence is present from penguins in the North Pole to babies in the Amazon. DDT, for example, has been discovered in the livers of ocean fish thousands of miles from where it was used for farming, as was noted by Dr. Jensen in his now-classic text *Empty Harvest*. "Deadly pesticides, like dioxin and PCB, now contaminate the entire food chain."[16]

Our only hope is that we have the necessary antidotes to some of their accumulated effects in the herbal kingdom. For hopeful new research in this area, see chapter 7.

If you are using artificial estrogen in combination with the xenoestrogens we are all bombarded with from the environment, you may be at much higher risk for cancer and other hormone-related disorders. There are many valuable natural estrogens in herbs. See the chart on herbs that balance hormones (page 323), and many excellent books on treating menopause, PMS, and other hormonal problems naturally.

Mad Cow and Related Diseases

Mad cow disease was discovered in 1985 when British cows started staggering around and dying. Autopsies showed their brains were full of sponge-like holes. A year later, Britain had an epidemic on its hands. In 1990, scientists noticed the similarity of mad cow in some human diseases, particularly one known in some primitive tribes as "ku-ku," which also eats holes in the brain and turns it to gelatin. Numerous species, from mink to sheep, now suffer a similar fate. What is going on that this ghastly disease is crossing species barriers?

Many scientists and environmentalists now believe we are fooling ourselves if we think that the practices that created the problem of mad cow disease (called, technically, bovine spongiform encephalopathy, or BSE) in Britain do not exist in the United States. Interestingly, the root of this terrifying problem, which has now spread into the human population, is a type of cannibalism. In other words, the cows become "mad" because they have developed a virus as a result of being fed rendered cow and sheep byproducts.

No doubt most Americans do not know (or would prefer *not* to know) that, despite the fact that there is now legislation to prohibit it, the feeding of cows to cattle is an ongoing practice in the United States. Howard Lyman of the Humane Society openly discussed the possibility that the disease may already exist in U.S. cattle on an Oprah Winfrey show in May of 1996. She was immediately hit with a food disparagement lawsuit, filed by Texas cattle owners. This kind of lawsuit is technically called SLAPPs, which stands for Strategic Lawsuit Against Public Participation. It was a hastily created suit designed to protect beef industry profits, and all Oprah was doing was discussing the risk factors of mad cow disease in the United States.

When the press shocked the world with the first deaths of people who had died of the human version of mad cow disease, called Creutzfeldt-Jakob Disease (CJD), little did anyone know that eating infected beef a whole decade earlier could cause such a tragedy. Then links started to unfold with those similar diseases in preliterate areas of the world that still practice a form of cannibalism, i.e., principally eating human brains of the deceased, which apparently was a religious practice. In one study of the Fore Highlanders of New Guinea, anthropologists traced the alarmingly high incidence of a terrible disease similar in many respects to mad cow but also resembling eubola, which is there called "laughing death," to this cannibalistic practice.[17] Links continued to unfold.

Peter Jennings did a news story on May 12, 1996, on the possibility of BSE-infected meat in the U.S. This was after a "voluntary ban" by the meat industry on March 30, 1996. The Jennings story disclosed that, in fact, the feeding of animal remains to livestock continues to be a widespread practice in this country. Are people dying of CJD in droves? CJD cannot spread from person to person except through transplants, hormone injections, and possibly blood transfusions. People catch the related disease from cows by eating cows contaminated with BSE or by taking drugs made from cow organs, bone meal from contaminated animals, and possibly growth hormones. ABC reported that health officials maintained that there are "only" 250 new cases of CJD in the United States every year.[18]

However, what is now diagnosed as Alzheimer's disease (and other forms of dementia)—which are certainly now attacking this country in great numbers in our elderly—may, in fact, be CJD or a form of it. As the ABC report went on to discuss, when pathologists examined brain tissue from patients with Alzheimer's and similar brain disorders, they uncovered hidden cases of CJD, which suggest, and I quote, that "a public health problem is being overlooked."[19] Given a very conservative estimate—say 1 percent of Alzheimer's patients with CJD—that would mean that there are 40,000 new cases a year. Remember, this disease has a latency period of up to forty years. Again, we may be seeing just the tip of the iceberg. Interestingly, the media is now beginning to focus on the onslaught of Alzheimer's in the baby boomer generation, focusing principally on how it may well make our health care system go bankrupt.

In February of 1998, Oprah beat the Big Beef case (thankfully demonstrating that freedom of speech in this country was not dead), but a CNN report assured the American public that there was absolutely no threat of mad cow in the U.S. from eating cows. Oprah was undaunted by the ordeal, as was Mr. Lyman, who said he still intends to champion food safety. By coincidence, the same week *Nova* did a special on mad cow, explaining that scientists are quite concerned about the problem (despite the reassurance of the main media).[20] BSE is indeed jumping the species barrier, as the report on Nova explained in detail. As it does so, scientists now believe, a frightening thing is happening: as the disease passes from one species to another, it becomes stronger, more virulent, and its incubation time appears to shrink. Then this new disease may be able to infect other species that were not previously susceptible to it. For example, we did not used to get scrapie from eating sheep, but cows got it, and humans got it from them. The alarming discovery is that now a *new* form of CDJ has been discovered, indicating a closer link to BSE. Scientists estimate that 18 million people in Britain, with a particular kind of genetic predisposition, may be at risk for this new form of CDJ if the current theory is correct: that CDJ is, in fact, a new form of BSE.[21]

The pathogen that causes BSE is confounding to researchers, because it is neither a virus nor a bacteria; it appears to be a type of protein. Thus, it does not behave like other pathogens: it cannot be killed by radioactivity, disinfectants, freezing, or any other known method. The chilling and very baffling mystery of the BSE pathogen is that it appears, somehow, to be immortal. The recent book *Deadly Feasts* is an excellent but frightening overview of this problem, with carefully documented evidence indicating how BSE and other animal diseases are, and may in the future, affect the human population.[22]

What is even more disconcerting is that the disease has not only crossed the species barrier but, like other forms of dementia, it can be inherited. In an article in *Scientific American* in 1995, where this problem was examined in depth, these diseases are lumped together and now called "prion diseases."[23] It has been discovered in cows, sheep, goats, pigs, and chickens. Even cats have been infected. In an on-line brief from the Green Group in the European Parliament in March of 1996, the point was made that since scientific studies have shown that the disease can be spread though feeding habits, it is up to us to exercise some measure of control. The Greens called for an end to mass assembly-line feeding of livestock and encouraged responsible humane methods of animal husbandry.

Perhaps the voice of nature is trying to tell us something. We should not be feeding animals other domesticated animals—especially from the same species—and then eating them. Perhaps we should not be eating them at all. Interestingly, the Bible tells us that human beings did not eat animals until the generation of Noah. Whether this is myth or dim recollection of history, the implications are intriguing. At any rate, it may be important to investigate the sources of meat you feed your children, and the sources upon which these animals feed.

Radiation and Toxic Waste

As far back as 1971, a presidential council warned about the dangers of electromagnetic radiation, which is now emanating from a number of places in our daily environment: TVs, computers, x-rays, microwaves, power lines, electric devices such as electric blankets, and food irradiation. Researchers have discovered that rats exposed to long-term low dosage microwave energy were four times as likely to develop malignant tumors.[24] Other studies have demonstrated that people regularly exposed to certain kinds of radiation—for example, power station operators and military personnel exposed to microwave radiation—had a three-fold increase in cancer than controls who were not regularly exposed.[25]

Radioactive isotopes can tend to accumulate in certain tissues in the body, especially the ovaries, testes, bowel, and skin. Others go directly to the bone and marrow, which is where many immune cells are produced. When immune cells are destroyed, the body is more vulnerable to invading pathogens that can cause disease. Since we are all exposed to some degree to environmental devices that may pose hazards to the immune system, it is essential to take daily doses of nutrients that will rebuild it. One major nutrient is ginseng. Another is blue-green algae. In the herbal kingdom, Irish moss and algae are the best supplements to counteract radioactivity in the body. Many natural seaweeds chelate out the toxic waste caused by radioactivity and some heavy metals (chelation is a process of removing heavy metals from the bloodstream; in nature, it is the combination of an organic compound with a metallic ion, which releases minerals for soil fertility; see chapter 3). Other immunostimulants listed in the herbal part of this book may be valuable as well.

The endocrine and immune systems are the part of the body most dependent on vitamins and minerals. Dr. Jensen, in his book *Empty Harvest*, has emphasized that iodine is one of the most important radiation protective factors.[26] Yet a daily intake of chlorine and sodium fluoride—which are added to most everyone's water supply without our permission—seriously inhibit the absorption of this essential nutrient. One marvels at the morality of imposing medication in our daily water intake without most people even being aware of it, especially when numerous studies have demonstrated the link between fluoride and toxicity.[27]

One serious danger about both fluoride and chlorine is that they are enzyme inhibitors. So if you have been exposed to radiation, it is vital to take iodine but useless to take it if you are drinking chlorinated and fluorinated water, since it destroys the potential for protein-bound iodine to be assimilated.

The Senate recently stopped the last hope that irradiated food be properly labeled, so we could have a choice at the supermarket. In December 1997, the FDA approved irradiation of meat, the last food to be approved. Aside from the fact that some people may not want to eat irradiated foods, the other no less serious problem this poses is that it demands that hundreds of new radiation plants be built, which creates a proliferation of radioactive materials in our environment, according to research from the University of California Newsletter.[28]

All proteins, fats, and enzymes are chemically altered when food is irradiated, and many now suspect that chromosome damage will result from the long-term effects of eating irradiated foods. Future generations may be the ones who suffer the most from this convenience, unless we continue to insist that we have a choice about the foods we buy at our local supermarkets.

Recycled Toxic Waste

We are all uncomfortably aware that there are pollutants in our environment in the form of chemicals and heavy metals, called, most frequently, "hazardous waste." Most Americans probably think it is tucked away in a silo someplace where, hopefully, it won't do *too* much harm. After all, what is the normal thing to do with a substance that is highly contaminated? It is to insulate it from the general population. What most of us are unaware of is that we have reached such a critical mass of toxic waste in our environment that we simply do not know what to do with it, and so one solution—which appears to border on the bizarre—is to recycle it back into our environment by spreading it on America's farmlands. True, most farmers don't know they are being duped into doing this. Nonetheless, it is becoming an alarming and widespread practice.

Geri Guidetti, who posts investigative reports regularly on her website called The Ark Institute, examined the numerous stories on this problem, which is now occurring with alarming frequency. Her report explained how excessive amounts of hazardous industrial wastes—including toxic heavy metals and radioactive substances—are being incorporated into fertilizers and then unwittingly applied to farmland throughout the United States.[29] Some horrendous examples—which are here given only to hint at the magnitude of this problem—include:

- Toxic waste is carried from Oregon steel mills to Washington, where it is stored in hazardous waste silos, then mixed with fertilizer. Washington is one of the principal places where much of America gets its apples.

- A uranium plant in Oklahoma is spraying grazing land with 10 million gallons of radioactive waste per year, which is called "liquid fertilizer." It is producing anomalies such as deformed cattle (one calf had two noses) and an increased incidence of cancer in people living in the area.

- In Georgia, toxic metal waste—lead, cadmium, and chromium—is mixed with zinc and sold as a fertilizer called LimePlus. These toxic ingredients are not listed on the label—they don't need to be. There is a lack of federal regulation and labeling requirements in this area, so many farmers do not even know that these new fertilizers contain these recycled toxic compounds. This particular formula was then discontinued because it killed a thousand acres of peanut crops. Farmers are left with the dilemma of trying to figure out how to get it out of their soils.

- A similar product, called NutriLime, is widely distributed in parts of the Pacific Northwest. It is principally from a chemical plant that is very high in lead, and the lead in the soil samples tested went from 4 parts per million to 562 parts per million after using the new fertilizer.

There is new evidence accumulating every day that points to the severity of this problem, but this should be enough to sound a wake-up call in the United States. Canada and Europe will not buy toxic industrial byproducts, which are now routinely spread on American farmlands, and there are limits set on lead and cadmium in their fertilizers. Not so in the United States, which, at the time of this writing, has no regulation yet in this area. In at least twenty-six states there are now programs that try to match hazardous waste generators with fertilizer "recyclers." "Why does it go on?" asks Ms. Guidetti. "Just because no one is watching? More than that: it's very profitable."[30]

The current situation with American farmers, to quote one "save the soil" activist by the name of Dieter Deumling, is that "they're constantly being frightened by chemical salesmen with the threat that if they abandon the use of what amounts to a whole medicine cabinet of chemical products, and turn to a more wholesome way of treating their land, they risk going broke, which they are doing anyway."[31]

Heavy metals do not go away, which is why the industries are so concerned with finding a way to recycle them. They accumulate in the environment and they accumulate in the human body. In areas where these products are being used, children who live there consistently show higher levels of lead, cadmium, arsenic, and aluminum than what is considered normal when hair samples were taken.[32] This is a very dangerous trend that must be monitored on a continued basis. As Ms. Guidetti explains,

> Mere trace amounts of lead can cause developmental defects in children. Lead in paint is regulated. Lead in gasoline is regulated. Lead in food cans is regulated. Lead in fertilizer is not regulated and is never disclosed on fertilizer labels even when it is found to be as high as three percent of the product. . . . How much toxic waste in our soils will finally amount to too much? Is there some unseen threshold we'll reach before we begin to see serious, irreversible problems?[33]

In 1980, the Surgeon General declared toxic waste sites an environmental emergency. In a research assessment report in 1985, it was revealed that there are nearly 10,000 hazardous waste sites that pose a serious threat to the public health of this country.[34] Altogether, there are now more than 375,000 sites, which is approximately 7,000 per state. This chemical avalanche is unlike anything else we have ever seen in human history. The effects are showing up in our health, and will continue to manifest in our children.

Symptoms of lead poisoning include nervousness, headaches, fatigue, muscular aches and pains, constipation, and, in serious cases, vomiting, anemia, chronic degenerative diseases, nerve damage, and brain dysfunction. According to one random study of more than 35,000 people, it was concluded that more than 40 percent of all U.S. children may have health problems due to lead poisoning.[35]

Cadmium toxicity includes symptoms such as kidney and liver damage, bronchitis, and suppressed T cell production. Studies are beginning to associate high levels of cadmium in people dying from disorders related to high blood pressure. Cadmium competes with zinc and when the body has an excess of cadmium, this valuable mineral is displaced. Adequate calcium, protein, iron, and zinc in your diet can help protect against cadmium absorption.

Aluminum and mercury are two other toxic chemicals that have infiltrated the food chain and that can cause any number of health hazards, from blurred vision and constipation to insanity and Alzheimer's disease. Dr. Alan Gaby has noted that of all the chemicals introduced into the environment this century, aluminum is the most prolific and one of the most dangerous. There are particularly strong doses of this metal in antacids, and Dr. Gaby warns that this ingested aluminum is implicated in osteoporosis.[36]

The best way to protect yourself and your family, of course, is to try and eat organic produce and dairy products, and wash all produce you are unsure of very well. Drink bottled or filtered water and maintain a holistic health regime as much as possible. In Steven Schechter's excellent book *Fighting Radiation and Chemical Pollutants with Foods, Herbs and Vitamins,* he lists a number of supplements to counteract the effects of some of these chemical toxins.[37] They include bee pollen; lecithin; chlorophyll; seaweeds; zinc; selenium; foods rich in pectin; fermented foods, especially yogurt and supplements like probiotics; and vitamins A, B, C, and E. The most powerful supplement, in my opinion, are the seaweed plants, particularly blue-green algae, spirulina, and Irish moss (see chapters 6 and 7 on antioxidants.)

Organic germanium holds great promise as an antimutagen and anticancer agent, and also has radioactive protective potential, especially if one is treated with radiation therapy. Studies show that, with the ingestion of germanium, radioactive rays are prevented from penetrating and destroying blood corpuscles and cells. The richest sources of organic germanium in the herbal kingdom are garlic and ginseng. New research also indicates that colloidal minerals may help flush toxic waste from the system. (More on this in the next chapter.) Informed consumers interested in following this story may want to check Ms. Guidetti's Ark Institute website (http://www.arkinstitute.com) or subscribe to *Rachel's Hazardous Waste News* from the Environmental Research Foundation.[38]

Genetically Engineered Foods

In 1994, the FDA approved the MacGregors tomato, which marked a major turning point in the development of food products that are the result of genetic engineering. The tomato was the result of $95 million of research and development. The technique had been perfected: code an enzyme involved in the ripening process and reverse it. It allows an extra five days for the tomato to ripen and therefore gives it an extended shelf life. The approval by the FDA marked a new onslaught of unknown risks to unsuspecting consumers. The law says it is not necessary for us to know, while wandering down the supermarket aisle, which fruits and vegetables have had their genes spliced and which have not.

It is becoming common practice to splice numerous plant, animal, even bacterial and viral genes in an attempt to alter plant growth rate, make processing easier and more profitable, and create more resistance to pests. Human genes have even been spliced into pigs, making them leaner. Companies are not required to label these products or reveal the source of the implanted genes.

Recombination is the exchange of parts of genes or blocks of genes between chromosomes. Pseudo-recombination is a similar process wherein gene components of a virus are exchanged with a protein coat of another. Most plants genetically altered for herbicide resistance use something called the cauliflower mosaic virus (CaMV). CaMV genes incorporated into the plant recombines with the infecting virus, a process questioned by a number of concerned scientists, who feel it is necessary to examine the safety of foods containing viral genes. One suspected outcome is that as large numbers of people eat CaMV modified foods, a recombination between CaMV and hepatitis B, a similar virus, will take place, creating, in effect, a supervirus that could thrive in plants, insects, and humans.[39]

There are other ways genetic foods may spread disease. In some tests, researchers found that when soybeans are modified with genes from Brazil nuts, it resulted in potentially deadly allergic reactions in people who could normally eat soybeans but not the nuts. People who are allergic to one type of food may suddenly discover their allergies now include many more foods. Some people can suffer distress or even fatal shock from eating peanuts, which are now present—in gene form—in some tomatoes.[40]

This is exactly the kind of problem that occurred with the tryptophan scandal. More than 1,500 people were permanently disabled and 37 died from this genetically manipulated product. Normally, tryptophan is a harmless food supplement, which was once on many health food store shelves. However, when Japanese genetic engineers altered the genetic material for tryptophan production to make it produce in much larger amounts, they caused it to also produce a powerful toxin. The genetic engineers had no idea that their tinkering had created this deadly contaminant until the supplement was marketed and people started dying. Because it was not labeled as genetically engineered, it took months to track down the source of the problem and remove the product from the market.[41]

Perhaps most frightening in terms of genetic manipulation of foods that guarantee our safely and livelihood is the Terminator model presently being developed by major seed companies, principally Monsanto, Delta, and Pine Land Co. The Terminator technology has benignly been called "Control of Plant Gene Expression," which essentially means that it permits the owners of these giant seed companies licenses to create sterile seed by selectively programming a plant's DNA to kill its own embryos. The result, of course, is that, if saved for future crops, the seed produced by these plants will not grow, thus forcing farmers to reinvest in seed every year from the developers of the Terminator. Another disturbing feature of this new technology is the deliberate disabling of natural plant functions that help fight disease, thus forcing farmers to buy more disease-fighting chemicals from the monstrous seed companies that sold them the seed in the first place. In her report on the Terminator, Ms. Guidetti has noted:

> [The] widespread global adoption of the newly patented Terminator Technology will ensure absolute dependence of farmers, and the people they feed, on multinational corporations for their seed and food. Dependence does not foster freedom. On the contrary, dependence fosters a loss of freedom. Dependence does not increase personal power, it diminishes it. . . . The Terminator Technology is brilliant science and arguably "good business," but it has crossed the line, the tenuous line between genius and insanity.[42]

Thankfully, Ms. Guidetti has created the Ark Institute, a resource for nonhybrid seed distribution, as an alternative to such madness.

Other dangers resulting from the practice of genetically altering foods are diminished nutritional quality, counterfeit freshness, and antibiotic resistance, as well as new environmental concerns. For example, crops engineered for herbicide resistance permit even more harmful chemicals to be sprayed onto these plants without killing them. This of course poses greater dangers for humans who consume the poisonous pesticides. It is speculated that this practice in America alone will increase the use of toxic chemicals three-fold, in a country where 80 percent of the ground water is already polluted by herbicides and other mutagenic agricultural chemicals.[43] In addition, another environmental hazard is the possibility that a gene inserted into a domesticated crop plant could spread to the wild, releasing genes to wild plants that then become herbicide resistant. Some scientists speculate that in ten to twenty years we could have a "superweed" catastrophe on our hands as a result of upsetting the intricate balance of nature. This could cause an immeasurable decrease in income from farm lands, not to mention the damage to our ecosystem.[44]

Then there are the religious and ethical issues. Some people may not care to eat vegetables with animal or human genes spliced into them. Genetically altered food threatens to sever the last remaining link between the foods that sustain life and Mother Nature herself.

Many scientists fear that genetically engineered organisms have already caused serious health problems in an unsuspecting population. Some believe it is yet another avenue for promoting cancer, by introducing greater amounts of toxins in our food and tearing down the body's immune response. Most disturbing, perhaps, is the fact that once introduced, organisms can never be recalled from the environment and their effects could spread without limit.

What can you do?

- Write the FDA Commissioner (HF-1, 5600 Fishers Lane, Rockville, MD, 20857) and demand federal policy on engineered foods with mandatory labeling.

- Contact your local supermarkets and school cafeterias; ask them to demand labeling. Or encourage them to ask their distributors to boycott known genetically engineered foods.

- Try to buy organic produce from local farmers whom you feel are consciously avoiding patented seeds from the biotech industry.

- Bless your food before you eat it and take herbal supplements daily to rid the body of excess poisons and strengthen the immune system.

Antibiotics and Infectious Diseases

In 1928, Sir Alexander Fleming's discovery of penicillin appeared to be the miraculous panacea that would vanquish infectious disease forever. When it works well, an antibiotic quells an infection by destroying the cell wall of the organism or by interfering with chemical messages essential for its reproduction. But over time, and through massive misuse and overuse of antibiotics, many disease-causing organisms have mutated; they have developed a stronger cell wall, changed their chemical messages, or by some other method have developed defense mechanisms to repel the once-lethal attack of the drug.

Numerous reports now indicate that antibiotics are frequently given to people without bacterial infections (which is the only kind of infection the drug is effective against) because patients are so demanding. So doctors hand over a prescription for a condition that they know will not work, many times for children. Since most patients don't know that antibiotics won't cure viruses or colds, it would appear that they need to be informed, rather than pacified. "Antibiotic pressure" is a lame excuse for doctors who know that by prescribing unnecessary drugs, the problem of antibiotic abuse and its consequences are only exacerbated.

A report was issued from the Center for Infectious Disease at the University of Texas–Houston Health Science Center indicating that the root of our present antibiotic resistance is overprescription, especially to children; widespread questionable use in hospitals; and drug misuse in Third World countries, where resistant bacteria continue to develop and are then imported into industrialized nations. For all practical purposes, it indicated that—from a scientific point of view—we may have reached the pinnacle of sophistication in our development of antibiotic drugs.[45]

The *FDA Consumer* warns that this antibiotic resistance is spreading rapidly. For example, in 1968, 12,5000 people in Guatemala died of an epidemic of shigella diarrhea because no antibiotic could destroy it. Deaths from pneumonia rose 12 percent between 1980 and 1985. Between 1979 and 1987, only 0.02 percent of pneumococcus strains infecting patients in this country were penicillin-resistant. In 1994, 6.6 percent of the same strains were resistant. There was a doubling in doctor's office visits for ear infections for preschoolers between 1975 and 1990, attributed to the increased use of day-care facilities. Many children are taken back for more prescriptions repeatedly because this has become one of the most difficult infections to effectively treat. In 1992, 13,000 hospital patients died of bacterial infections that were resistant to antibiotic treatment. Between 1983 and 1990, all E. coli strains tested were killed by antibiotics. By 1993, only 11 of 40 tested strains of this deadly disease were resistant.[46]

According to a report in the April 28, 1994, issue of the *New England Journal of Medicine*, researchers have now identified bacteria that resist all antibiotic drugs currently available.[47] This becomes even more frightening when one considers the fact that in some places scientists are testing the limits of such formidable threats as eubola or anthrax for potential use in biological warfare. In August of 1997, it was revealed that the U.S. was funding secret biological laboratories in Russia. The Defense Department spokesman said, "We're trying to keep them at the lab bench. We're concerned about the proliferation problem."[48] Purportedly, Russian scientists have already developed a genetically modified strain of anthrax that resists all vaccines and antibiotics known today. When the strange tale emerged of two men arrested in Las Vegas in February, 1998, claiming to have enough anthrax to wipe out the entire city, it gave Americans across the nation reason to pause. It did not help knowing that it turned out to be a nonlethal form of anthrax. It brought to everyone's attention how dangerously easy such biological weapons are to produce.[49]

As fears of Y2K increased across the nation in 1999, so did the concern among top government officials that this weakened condition could make us extremely vulnerable to threats of biological and chemical terrorism. Although there is not much we can do about the nature of this threat, we can certainly raise our awareness about the abuse of antibiotics and the rapid deterioration its use has on the immune system; we can also continue to take personal responsibility for building strong immune systems in ourselves and our children through the use of herbal supplementation. In major world disasters, the strong survive. Obviously, in order to build a healthy immune system in today's world, one needs to be continually vigilant.

Another major concern, in terms of antibiotic abuse, is the overuse of antibiotics in livestock, where they are used in huge quantities to "prevent disease." If an animal has an infection, it does not put on weight as quickly and is not worth as much. The real reason for this blatant abuse—when animals are fed antibiotics over long duration—is to convert animal feed to profitable units of animal food. Poultry is a prime problem area. The practice of feeding chickens these drugs, according to *Harvard Women's Health Watch* magazine, "turns these animals into a breeding ground for resistant bacteria. We ultimately consume these pathogens along with the meat on our tables."[50] Cases have now been documented where people have developed multi-drug resistant salmonella food poisoning after consuming beef from cows fed large amounts of antibiotics. What continued use of this practice will ultimately do to our immune systems is something I would not care to guess at.

Unfortunately, antibiotics are not only fed to livestock. They are also disseminated in waterways for fish. According to one report, "Antibiotics used in farming and aquaculture have resulted in multi-drug resistant pathogen contaminated foods which produce infections in consumers. Multi-drug resistance is both a local and global health hazard of epidemic proportions."[51] We need only remember that a new strain of flu virus killed 25 million people around the world in the early part of this century before it was brought under control. It attacked one out of every two people.

One spokesman for the Center for Infectious Disease in Houston has said, "I think we've gone about as far as we can go in terms of developing new antibiotics. In the future, we will see more focus on the patient and ways to boost the patient immune system and resistance to infection."[52] This, of course, is the philosophy that holistic practitioners have been proposing for decades. The role of food supplements in fortifying the body against infection has not generally been embraced by traditional medicine. But that does not prevent researchers from all over the world from presenting their many findings about the immune-building aspects of vitamins, minerals, antioxidants, and other nutritional supplements, including vitally important enzymes.

The Catch-22 with antibiotics is that they kill all manner of bacteria without discrimination, and when we kill friendly bacteria in the body—the microflora in the intestines, for example—we undermine the immune system even more. The reason many people get diarrhea or upset stomachs when they take antibiotics is because every possible protective bacteria in the gut is destroyed, leading to all kinds of enzyme imbalances. For example, antibiotics destroy the friendly bacteria that produce vitamin B12, which maintains the health of the red blood cells that are so important for life.

According to the holistic model, when we have some kind of invading infection, it is not the fault solely of the germ; it is because the immune system has been undermined and cannot fight it. To believe totally in the "germ theory" of disease is to think in a way that is very similar to our unenlightened ancestors, who thought that demons or curses were the cause of disease. Today we still tend to project the evil presence outside, only now we call it "germs." Without undermining the value of good sanitation, the first alternative we should examine is our attitude. Instead of viewing disease as an attack of something evil, we should ask: What is the essentially good presence that is missing? What is lacking nutritionally that makes the body disease-resistant, as it should be? Where there is malnourished, enzyme-depleted tissue, there is the opportunity for bacteria and viruses, which are cell scavengers, to invade. Our job, perhaps, is to keep the inner house clean.

Of course a balance needs to be struck here. If the germs—our modern demons—are mutating and getting stronger, we need to compensate by creating even healthier immune systems. It continually amazes me how little most of us do on a daily basis to insure that this is accomplished. Often people come to me (and herbalists around the world, I'm sure) with a complaint, and expect a miracle herbal cure overnight.

Although we need to acknowledge the shadow element in what we have unleashed in our environment and attempt to rectify it, we must not feel victimized by it, because with consistent inquiry we can discover the missing element that can enable us to create homeostasis once again. Of this I feel certain. And I am convinced many of our most powerful allies will come from the plant kingdom. Recent studies have suggested that time-honored supplements, like echinacea and Saint John's Wort, are valuable in protecting us from infections and maintaining a healthy immune response. Other excellent immune-building herbs are garlic, ginseng, and cat's claw. (See the chart on antioxidant and immunostimulant herbs [page 321] and the discussion in chapters 6 and 7.) Amazingly, we are discovering new immunostimulants in the herb kingdom continually.

Healing plants include not only herbs but foods. Diet and supplements may be the single most important tool for bringing health and balance back into our lives. In 1988, the U.S. Surgeon General's Report estimated that two-thirds of all deaths in the U.S. were diet-related. One of the most enlightened researchers in this area, Dr. Royal Lee, said nearly thirty years ago that "one of the biggest tragedies of human civilization is the precedence of chemical therapy over nutrition. It's a substitution of artificial therapy over natural, of poisons over food, in which we are feeding people poisons (drugs), trying to correct the reactions of starvation."[53]

There are so many nutrients in the herb and plant kingdom that are immune-building that I am not going to examine them in more detail here. They are listed in various places in this book. The bigger question at the moment is: Why are we starving?

Notes

1. Interview with Dr. Lynn Goldman, E.P.A. Office of Prevention, Pesticides & Toxic Substances, Associated Press release in *San Francisco Chronicle*, 7 June 1996, "With Pesticides 1 Plus 1 Sometimes Equals 1000."

2. M. S. Compton, *Women At the Change: An Intelligent Woman's Guide to Menopause* (St. Paul, MN: Llewellyn Publications, 1997).

3. J. Jacobson, et al., "Prenatal experience to an environmental toxin: A test of the multiple effects model," *Developmental Psychology* 20 (1984): 523–532.
   See also: J. Jacobson, et al., "A four year follow-up study of children born to consumers of Lake Michigan fish," *Journal of Great Lakes Research* 19 (1989): 776–783.

4. E. Carlson, et al., "Evidence for decreasing quality of semen during past 50 years," *British Medical Journal* 304 (1992): 609–613. See also J. Raloff, "The Gender Benders," *Science News* 145 (8 January 1994): 24–27; and R. M. Sharpe and N. E. Skakkaback, "Are estrogens involved in falling sperm counts and disorders of the male reproductive tract?" *The Lancet* 341 (1993): 1392–1395.

5. In J. Starrels, "Hand-Me-Down-Poisons," *The Green Guide* (14 July 1997), p. 1.

6. T. Colborn, D. Dumanoski, and J. P. Myers, *Our Stolen Future* (New York: Dutton, 1996).

7. Starrels, pp. 2–3.

8. Ibid.

9. L. S. Birnbaum, "Endocrine Effects of Prenatal Exposure to PCBs, Dioxins, and Other Xenobiotics: Implications for Policy and Future Research," *Environmental Health Perspectives* 102 (1994): 676–679. See also H. J. Pluim, et al., "Effects of Dioxins on Thyroid Function in Newborn Babies," *The Lancet* 339 (1992): 1303.

10. Compton, *Women at the Change,* e.g., see the last chapter with the interview with Dr. John Lee.

11. D. Davis, H. Bradlow, M. Wolff, T. Woodruff, D. Hoel, and H. Anton-Culver, "Medical Hypothesis: Xeno-Estrogen as Preventable Causes of Breast Cancer," *Environmental Health Perspectives* 101, no. 5 (1993): 372–377. See also D. Hunter and K. Kelsey, "Pesticide Residue and Breast Cancer: The Harvest of a Silent Spring?" *Journal of the National Cancer Institute* 85, no. 8 (1993): 598–599.

12. M. Wolff, P. Toniolo, E. Lee, M. Rivera, and N. Dubin, "Blood Levels of Organochlorine Residues and Risk of Breast Cancer," *Journal of the National Cancer Institute* 85, no. 8 (1993): 648–652. See also P. Pujol, S. Hilsenbeck, G. Chamness, and R. Elledge, "Rising Levels of Estrogen Receptor in Breast Cancer Over 2 Decades," *Cancer* 74, no. 5 (1994): 1601–1606; and S. Rier, D. Martin, R. Bowman, W. Dmowski, and J. Becker, "Endometriosis in Rhesus Monkeys Following Chronic Exposure to 2,3,7,8-Tetrachlorodibenzo-p-Dioxin," *Fundamental and Applied Toxicology* 21 (1993): 433–441.

13. A. M. Soto, et al., "The pesticides endosulfan, toxaphene, & dieldrin have estrogenic effects on human estrogen-sensitive cells," *Environmental Health Perspectives* 102 (1994): 380–383; and G. Greene, et al., "Can environmental estrogens cause breast cancer?" *Scientific American* (20 June 1994): 166–172.

14. T. A. Mably, et al., "In utero & lactational exposure of male rats to 2, 3, 7, 8 Tetrachlorodibenzo-P-dioxin," *Toxicology & Applied Pharmacology* 114 (May 1992): 97–126; and J. Raloff, "Perinatal dioxin feminizes male rats," *Science News* 141 (30 May 1992): 359.

15. In a presentation by Julia Langer, director of Wildlife Toxicology Program at WWF Canada, an on-line report, "Special Session for Journalists on Endocrine Disruptors," 17 February 1998. See also the WWF Science Unit in Washington, D.C., which has an extensive database of over 12,000 papers, many of which address endocrine-related disorders.

16. B. Jensen and M. Anderson, *Empty Harvest* (Garden City Park, NY: Avery Publishing Group, 1990), p. 12.

17. Nova report, "The Brain Eater," BBC/WGBH (Boston) co-production, February 1998.

18. ABC-TV World News Tonight, 12 May 1996.

19. Ibid.

20. Nova report.

21. Ibid.

22. R. Rhodes, *Deadly Feasts* (New York: Simon & Schuster, 1997).

23. S. B. Prusiner, "The Prion Diseases," Scientific American 272, no. 1 (January 1995): 48–57.

24. S. Schechter, *Fighting Radiation & Chemical Pollutants with Foods, Herbs, and Vitamins* (New York: Vitality Ink Publishers, 1992), pp. 33 and 15.

25. Ibid.

26. B. Jensen and M. Anderson, *Empty Harvest*.

27. G. L. Waldbott, "Fluoridation of community water supplies," *Journal of Allergy & Clinical Immunology* 48 (1971): 253–254 (letter). Also see his *Fluoridation, the Great Dilemma* (Lawrence, KS: Coronado Press, 1978). For early research in this area, see also W. L. Ledbeck, et al., "Acute sodium fluoride poisoning," *Journal of American Medical Association* 121 (1943): 826–827. See also the more recent research on the negative relationship between fluoride and bone loss: L. R. Hedlund, et al., "Increased incidence of hip fracture in osteoporotic women treated with sodium fluoride," *Journal of Bone & Mineral Research* 4 (1989): 223–225.

28. *University of California Wellness Newsletter*, "Our Beef with Irradiation," 14, no. 6 (March 1998): 3.

29. G. Guidetti, "America's Farmlands Are New Hazardous Waste Dumps," 26 July 1997. On-line report at The Ark Institute (http://www.arkinstitute.com). Ark Institute, P.O.B. 142, Oxford, OH, 45056.

30. Ibid.

31. P. Tomkins and C. Bird, *Secrets of the Soil* (New York: Harper & Row, 1989), p. 204.

32. Schechter, *Fighting Radiation*, p. 36.

33. Guidetti, *America's Farmlands*.

34. Schechter, *Fighting Radiation*, p. 36.

35. Ibid, p. 39.

36. A. Gaby, *Preventing and Reversing Osteoporosis* (Rocklin, CA: Prima Pub., 1994), pp. 191–218.

37. S. Schechter, *Fighting Radiation & Chemical Pollutants with Foods, Herbs and Vitamins* (New York: Vitality Ink Publishers, 1992).

38. The Ark Institute (www.arkinstitute.com). Ark Institute, P.O.B. 142, Oxford, OH, 45056. See also Environmental Research Foundation, P.O.B. 5036, Annapolis, MD, 21403.

39. On-line report, J. E. Cummins, "The Use of the Cauliflower Mosaic Virus 35S Promoter (CaMV) in Calgene's Flavr Savr Tomato Creates Hazard," unpublished paper dated 3 June 1994. Dr. Cummins is associate professor of genetics in the department of plant sciences at the University of Western Ontario in London, Ontario.

40. J. Fagan, *Genetic Engineering: The Hazards; Vedic Engineering: The Solutions* (Fairfield, IA: MIU Press, 1995). See also H. R. Hill, "OSU study finds genetic altering of bacterium upsets natural order," *The Oregonian* (8 August 1994); and M. Wadman, "Genetic resistance spreads to consumers," *Nature* 383 (October 1996): 564.

41. J. Fagan, "Genetically Engineered Foods—Good For Our Planet?" *Explorer* 8 (1997): 3–5.

42. G. Guidetti, "Seed Terminator and Mega-Merger Threaten Food and Freedom," on-line report, 5 June 1998, The Ark Institute (www.arkinstitute.com). Ark Institute, P.O.B. 142, Oxford, OH, 45056.

43. J. Fagan, " Genetically Engineered . . . ," p. 3.

44. T. Mikkelson, et al., "The risk of crop transgene spread," *Nature* 380 (October 1996): 31; and J. Kling, "Could transgenic supercrops one day breed superweeds?" Science 274, no. 11 (October 1996): 180–181.

45. On-line report, R. Calligaris, "Are antibiotics losing their power?" UT Lifetime Health Letter (September 1994). See also S. Begley, "The End of Antibiotics?" *Newsweek* 123 (7 March 1994): 47–52; and J. Travis, "Reviving the Antibiotic Miracle?" *Science* 264 (15 April 1994): 360–362.

46. On-line report, R. Lewis, "The rise of antibiotic infections," *FDA Consumer* 29, no. 7 (September 1997).

47. *New England Journal of Medicine*, quoted in Lewis, above.

48. Quoted in the *San Francisco Examiner*, Sunday, 10 August 1997, p. A3, "U.S. Funding Biological Labs in Russia."

49. Reported in the *Seattle Times*, 18 February 1998; CNN News; and numerous other places.

50. *Harvard Women's Health Watch* 4, no. 8 (April 1997): 3; See also M. Sun, "Antibiotics and animal feed: a smoking gun," *Science* 225 (21 September 1984): 1375; E. Marshall, "Scientists endorse ban on antibiotics in feeds," *Science* 222 (11 November 1983): 601; J. C. Juskevich, et al., "Bovine Growth Hormone: Human Food Safety Evaluation," *Science* 249 (1990): 877.

51. On-line report, "Antibiotic Resistance," Bug Bytes 2, no. 13 (4 October 1995): 2. A production of LSU Medical Center, Shreveport.

52. Calligaris, p. 2.

53. B. Jensen and M. Anderson, *Empty Harvest: Understanding the Link Between our Food, Our Immunity, and Our Planet* (Garden City Park, NY: Avery Publishing Group, 1990), p. 106.

*So long as one feeds on food from unhealthy soil, the spirit will
lack the stamina to free itself from the prison of the body.*
—RUDOLF STEINER

3

Our Devastated Soil and the Magic That's Missing

Many people would no doubt agree that there are grave dangers connected to our reckless use of pesticides and preservatives, which are foreign substances to the body that previous generations were never exposed to. However, in the past few years, attention has refocused on the rising incidence health problems caused by the "mineral factors." Our mineral-depleted topsoil has alarmed so many that the vast majority of health and nutrition experts agree that, even though we may eat three large meals a day, we are starving at the cellular level. One study, which can be found in Senate Document 264, states:

> The alarming fact is that fruits, vegetables and grains now being raised on millions of acres of land that no longer contain enough of certain minerals are starving us—no matter how much of them we eat. . . . No man today can eat enough fruits and vegetables to

supply his system with the minerals he requires for perfect health because his stomach isn't big enough to hold them.[1]

This is a sad state of affairs and it continues to worsen every day. In addition, the protein content of our foods is only a fraction of what it used to be. For example, the protein content of wheat, once as much as 40 percent, is now only 13 or 14 percent. Most people in the U.S. are unaware that, even with the consumption of meat, there is a strong possibility of severe amino acid deficiency, animals eat the grain that is now so nutrient-poor.

Numerous scientists and doctors believe that there is a relationship between these deficiencies and such conditions as learning disabilities, addictions, food binges, depressions, degenerative diseases, and the weakening of our immune systems. Dr. Linus Pauling, winner of two Nobel Prizes, believed that most every sickness and ailment can be traced to a mineral deficiency. Our modern diet is only a shadow of the healthy diet that it once was, and the mineral legacy in our soil that has taken thousands of years to create has disappeared in a generation. So often when a body pain or other problem arises the first thing we think of is relieving the effects or symptoms of the malfunction. Rarely do we think about the possible underlying causes, so anxious are we to get relief. We are an instant gratification generation, and we must now look at what is causing our problems . . . or suffer the consequences.

It is quite obvious by now that insecticides do not do the job they were designed for; in fact, they simply breed larger numbers of more resistant bugs, in the same way that our overuse of antibiotics has. Not only do they poison our ecosystem, but the crops produced are no longer healthy. Crop loss continues to rise because the fruits and vegetables sprayed become more vulnerable to attack. Yet, as far back as 1940, concerned soil ecologists and agriculturists demonstrated that plant vulnerability to insects and fungus was caused by chemical toxicity and lack of real nutrition in a mineral-deficient soil. Unfortunately, crops grown on depleted soils produce malnourished bodies, upon which all manner of diseases can prey. Dr. D. W. Cavanaugh, of Cornell University, put it bluntly: "There is only one major disease and that is malnutrition."[2]

The main nutrients that we get from chemical fertilizers are the scientific trinity called NPK (nitrogen, phosphorus, and potassium). Since it was discovered that plants fed only these minerals could survive and look reasonably good, the Big Three have been aggressively marketed to U.S. farmers. Never mind that the human body needs seventy plus minerals for optimum health. Perhaps when this formula was first designed, at the turn of the century, information about good nutrition was lacking. But by the time we discovered the importance of these missing minerals, this farming practice had become big business. And when it comes to business versus health, it's always the same political battlefield, with money coming out on top. As Dr. Jensen, who wrote the book *Empty Harvest*, said, "The first thing to overcome is the mentality of our addiction to chemicals and their poisoned promises."[3]

Dr. Jensen and others have pointed out that we could easily put these desperately needed minerals back into our soils by feeding them organic humus, seaweed fertilizers, and rock dust, such as the glacial mink used by the Hunza people, or colloidal soft rock, a mineral food found on several places of our planet in great abundance.[4] It is part mineral from volcanic ash and part mineral from calciferous bodies of marine algae. Mineralogists sometimes refer to it as rhyolite; other use it interchangeably with bentonite. As explained by Peter Tompkins,

> [G]eologists consider it to be an ancient oceanic deposit brought to the surface by volcanic action, a form of heavy sedimentation on the sea floor, a mixture of mineral elements and marine life such as seaweed, shrimp, and algae. The clay contains all the essential trace minerals in a balanced ratio, as laid down by nature. In this form the minerals are naturally chelated, as in plants and animals, in an organic, easily assimilable form.[5]

It is crucial that we feed our soils if we are to successfully survive into the next century. Soil without humus is dead. The alternative, if this is not done on a massive scale, is continued erosion and increased

chronic and acute diseases. The other possibility, for many nutrition-
ists investigating other alternatives on a less global, more individual
level, is to consume these nutrients directly, in the form of dense
green chlorophyll foods and colloidal minerals. This is what many
thousands of people are now doing.

The phenomenal health of the Hunzas (they have virtually no
"modern" degenerative diseases and most live to be over 100) has
been traced to the finely powdered debris of rock made by huge glac-
iers grinding down the side of the Himalayas, collecting silt, and slid-
ing into pools and rivers, where it is considered to be the healthiest
water for drinking. Because of its pearly gray color, it is called "glacial
milk," and when tourists visit there, they are often offered a more
"clear" water from their wells as a gesture of politeness. However, the
Hunza always drink their gray colloidal rock water themselves
because they know it is part of the healthy magic of their paradise.

Albert Schatz, who discovered the antibiotic streptomycin, also
first discovered what chelation is and how it works as a principle
chemical mechanism in the formation of soil fertility. He observed
how lichens, a form of algae, clung to and eventually decomposed
rock by literally eating it away. The lichens were chelating the rock to
extract its minerals.

This continued weathering process is what then releases minerals
for the growth of new plants. He was intrigued that in some places
where people seem to live longest and be most healthy, such as the
Incas near Machu Picchu or the Hunzas of the Himalayas, the soil
conditions were extremely rich in nutrients. They had developed successful agriculture without chemicals because they used an extremely
well-composted humus rich in a plant substance that, like lichen, dissolves minerals in the soil. It does this by putting minerals in a
chelated or colloidal condition, thus making every possible nutrient
available to the plant. In the case of the Incas, the "magical" herb was
called "harakkeh'ama;" it was even used to soften the rock that the
Incas used to build their huge monuments at Machu Picchu. It is
only through this process of chelation that bacteria are able to thrive
in the soils, making it fruitful. Bacteria (the friendly kind) are seldom

present in dying soils. One of the secrets of Hunza health is that they never plow deep because it submerges bacteria vital to the topsoil. Soil without humus and without bacterial action is not really alive; numerous soil experts agree that the reason the bacteria in the soil fail to function properly is because of the lack of natural trace elements and catalysts.

Dr. Schatz tried desperately to convince U.S. agriculturalists of the importance of using humus with chelating properties in 1963, when he published his work. But by then no one was interested. The NPK trinity was the king of the hour, and using old-fashioned humus seemed like an impractical thing to do. Little did the farmers of that decade know how many of us, three decades later, would wake up to the vital necessity of reclaiming the full spectrum of colloidal minerals and trace minerals in our daily diets.

An excellent book that examines alternatives to soil depletion is *Secrets of the Soil* by Peter Tompkins and Christopher Bird. They interviewed a geological prospector, Rollin Anderson, who mines mineral-rich rock soil in Utah. He summed up the problem when he said,

> We have ganged up on nature by taking the attitude that insects are invading our fields and destroying our crops. So we kill the bugs, thinking it correct. Instead we are killing ourselves. But the bugs are only destroying our crops because we are not feeding the crops their proper food.[6]

For people like Anderson, colloidal mineral food is the element necessary to correct the imbalances caused by foods that now contain only three minerals.

Colloidal soft rock phosphates promote the electrical properties in soil to activate release of its elements. For example, sticky clay soils become loose healthy soil when colloidal soft rock is added. Most of it comes from non-limestone, ocean vertebrate deposits in the earth, which need to be mined. Dr. Jensen explains that an unusual property of colloidal soft rock is that it keeps the minerals near the top of the plant, instead of gravitating into deeper layers of the soil, thus retarding erosion, increasing water retention, and feeding healthy bacteria. Colloids are the pantry in which the plant nutrients are stored and released over time as needed. It is a well-known fact that vegetables high in mineral content will look and taste better, be more resistant to disease and frost, and of course, be much more nutritious. In his review of this problem, Dr. Jensen has said, "I know of no method more capable of rapid remineralization of our crop lands, pasture and forests than the 'rock dust' method."[7]

The principal key to healthy vegetables is not nitrates; it is trace minerals. A pioneer in this area is Dr. Melchior Dikkers, professor of Biochemistry and Organic Chemistry at Loyola University, who claims that trace minerals are the key to all living organisms and essential to the metabolism of every living creature. He believes that colloidal soft rock is one of the most amazing sources of trace minerals he has ever examined.[8]

Colloidal soft rock typically forms microscopic, or at least very small, platy micaceous crystals. When water is absorbed by the crystals they tend to swell to several times their original volume. This is part of colloidal magic. It slows the progress of water through rocks and soil and prevents leakage of toxic fluids from attacking the roots of the plant. One way of decontaminating radioactive water is by slurring it with mineral clay. Likewise, clays like bentonite have been proven to absorb radioactivity in the body. Clay works against radioactivity because it has a negative effect on the ionized radioactive particles taken into the body. It may absorb a number of other harmful contaminants as well. Actually, according to Daniel Mowrey (*The Scientific Validation of Herbal Medicine*) it is not "absorbent"—rather, bentonite and similar clays are "adsorbent." He explains, "[I]t is capable of adsorbing many times its weight and volume in an aqueous medium."[9]

The difference between absorption and adsorption is a subtle but important one. Absorption occurs when substances are sucked into the internal structure of other substances, such as cells. Adsorption requires only that substances stick to the outside of the medium to which they are attracted. This means that the two substances retain their separate ionic charges, i.e., they have opposite electrical charges.

Minerals in a colloidal form have a predominately negative charge, which attracts to itself many positive electrical particles.

This has particular importance for allergens, according to Mowrey's research, because colloids quickly neutralize allergens before they invade the blood cells, i.e., the adsorptive surfaces prevent the allergic reaction.

Whenever colloidal rock phosphates are worked into the soil, plants thrive and become disease resistant without the use of any kind of pesticide. This is because, as explained before, colloids are the pantry of the plant kingdom. There is a lot of interest in —and confusion about—what colloidal mineral substances are. Colloidal is a condition, not a mineral. According to Tompkins and Bird, in *Secrets of the Soil,*

> [F]ine dust-like particles pass into the colloidal state of fineness upon reaching a critical size when their activity prevents them from settling out as molecules of their particular inorganic element . . . those materials which readily crystallize have the vital function of diffusing readily through animal membranes, as opposed to amorphous masses, which do not diffuse readily or at all through animal membranes, and cannot therefore be assimilated.[10]

According to the law of physics, the smaller an element is divided, the larger the surface mass it can cover; and the larger the surface area exposed, the more charged with energy the particle becomes. Wolfgang Pauli, the famous Nobel laureate, came to the conclusion after studying colloids that they are the most important link between organic and inorganic life.

To explain this in layman's terms: Although a human being cannot eat a nail, the iron can be absorbed if it is in a chelated or colloidal form (as in supplements). If the nail is converted into very fine steel wool, the surface-to-mass ratio becomes very large. Now, we should not go around eating steel wool, of course! However, this illustrates the difference between a mineral in a dense inorganic state and a state where its weight has been distributed over more mass. In the latter case, it is more readily available to release energy. One can put a match to a mass of very fine steel wool and it will catch on fire; its surface-to-mass ratio is so large (and its particles so small) that it is easily converted into another form of energy. This similar chemical effect occurs in the human body when we "burn" food. The smaller the particle, the more available it is for its enzyme activity to be utilized in the body.

One reason colloids are fast being recognized as an important food supplement is not only that they replace the minerals of our impoverished soils. It has been discovered that they allow for the maximum absorption of nutrients from food. Normally, nutrients carried by the bloodstream tend to be blocked from reaching the cells by pollutants stored in the connective tissue. The nutrients must literally fight their way through these contaminated tissues, often with little or no success. Like many herbs, colloidal minerals help attract and flush out these pollutants, thus allowing greater assimilation of nutrients from foods and food supplements. They also enhance the body's production of enzymes.

The importance of enzymes cannot be emphasized enough. Dr. Edward Howell, the father of modern enzyme research, has written that enzyme deficiency is a significant cause of premature aging and the development of numerous degenerative diseases.[11] Trace minerals are necessary for the creation of enzymes. Enzymes are destroyed by heat (cooking over 118 degrees), fluorine, chlorine, lead, nicotine, nitrates, pesticides, and chemical fertilizers. Since many of us are exposed to one or more of these life-destroying agents daily, it is imperative that we supplement our diets with enzymes and colloidal trace minerals. Once the supply of enzymes is depleted, life ceases. It does not matter how many vitamins we take, either, as vitamins are completely useless without enzymes.

In the philosophy of the great herbalist, Dr. John Christopher (to be examined more in upcoming chapters), vitamin and mineral supplements, because they are fractionated (that is, isolated from the way in which they occur in nature), should be treated as toxic waste in the body. Minerals, in an unnatural form, in particular, can accumulate and cause harmful effects. Yet clearly we need minerals today as never before, because of our impoverished soils. Most supplements only offer a few of the many essential nutrients necessary to sustain good health. But most colloidal mineral supplements replenish these needed seventy plus minerals once they have been stabilized in a liquid form. I do not recommend products such as montmorillonite, which contain too many inorganic rock elements to be easily digested or assimilated by the body. According to David Christopher, at the School for Natural Healing in Utah, minerals should come solely from the plant kingdom, such as jurassic greens and wheat grass.[12]

Others feel that colloidal minerals should be hydrophilic, or water soluble, which is what causes them to work with, not against, the body's natural process of assimilation. The best colloidal supplements, in my opinion, are from companies that have used deposits from ancient rainforests and marine life, such as those from the T. J. Clark mines in Utah. These are mined from mineral-rich vegetation sources that are plant-derived and negatively ionized. It is fine to feed colloidal soft rock to plants, which can then use the minerals and convert it into a form the body can use, but I don't advise eating rocks to get minerals. One researcher jokingly said, "People taking some of these inorganic metallic mineral products are going to have trouble getting through an airport metal detector."[13]

Many blue algae products (available in most drug stores), both from the sea and cultivated in some mineral-rich lakes, also contain most of the essential trace minerals. These minerals are called "essential" because they are! I want to emphasize again that vitamin supplements are useless without these vital minerals, something I did not know for years.

When we return to the practice of feeding our soils colloidal soft rock, our soils will begin to nourish us properly again. This practice, according to Rollin Anderson, helps to satisfy the soil's hidden hunger and correct the depletion of minerals over long periods of time.[14]

We all suffer this hidden hunger, a consequence of our ravaging of Mother Earth. Thankfully, she has still left us some hidden reserves and the magic that is missing is still available, waiting only for our discovery. Let's hope we find it in time.

Notes

1. "Farm Land Mineral Depletion: Senate Document #264" (1936), 74th Congress, 2nd Session.

2. Quoted in B. Jensen and M. Anderson, *Empty Harvest: Understanding the Link Between our Food, Our Immunity, and Our Planet* (Garden City Park, NY: Avery Publishing Group, 1990), p. 8.

3. Jensen, p. 102.

4. Ibid.

5. P. Tompkins and C. Bird, *Secrets of the Soil* (New York: Harper & Row, 1989), p. 216.

6. Ibid., pp. 224–225.

7. Jensen, p. 81.

8. Tompkins, p. 220.

9. D. Mowrey, *The Scientific Validation of Herbal Medicine* (New Canaan, CT: Keats Pub., Inc., 1986), pp. 130–131.

10. Tompkins, p. 222.

11. E. Howell, *Enzyme Nutrition: The Food Enzymes Concept* (Wayne, NJ: Avery Publishing Group, 1986).

12. David Christopher, personal phone conversation, 10 February 1998.

13. On-line report: Technical bulletin, Robert Musack, president, C & M Laboratories, Inc., 1 May 1996.

14. Tompkins, p. 216.

In order to conceptualize drugs as materials for restoring balance, the scientific world will have to undergo a total paradigm shift.

—Dr. Daniel Mowrey, author,
"Scientific Validation of Herbal Medicine"

4

The Only Solution Left

*A*merican health has degenerated in direct proportion to our departure from nature over the past century. America was the healthiest country in the world between 1900 and 1940, according to the U.S. Public Health Service. Our elders who lived before World War II know that our fruits, vegetables, and grains bear no resemblance to what they were before the war. Although crop yields may have increased, nutritive quality has progressively decreased—and with it, our overall health. Since 1945, we have had an explosion of degenerative diseases in this country, rising sharply by 60 percent.[1] Our discussion in the last chapter leads to the inevitable conclusion that America needs to look at alternative agriculture and healing methods if we want to return to the healthy nation we used to be.

There is a growing consciousness in both the educated public and in research scientists today concerning the importance of returning to plant-based nutritional supplements and herbs. In 1992, the National Institute of Health established the Office of Alternative Medicine to explore the promising benefits of nontraditional forms of medicine such as herbal healing. In the next few chapters, I want to explore the importance of using phytonutrients, especially from the herbal kingdom, as well as examine some of the cautions about their use. I would also like to paint a brief sketch of the three major herbalists who have influenced me over the past twenty years or so, because I am indebted to them for the many healing experiences I have witnessed in my life and in the lives of many others.

Some people write whole books surveying the grave health dangers and ecological disasters that plague our modern society. In researching the major dangers in our food supply and environment in the last two chapters, I did not want to paint a picture that is so bleak, it leaves one feeling hopeless. On the contrary, we must become a solution-oriented generation if we and our children are going to successfully survive into the next century. If one in eight school-age children in the U.S. have blood pressure levels that are considered high enough to be unhealthy for their age, and if obesity in children under age ten jumped more than 50 percent in the past two decades (both true), then we need to focus on workable solutions to these growing problems.[2] Part of the problem with obesity, as we have seen, is an internal hunger for missing nutrients. This is the legacy our next generation is inheriting. It is our first responsibility to protect the children. In addition, we must have positive reasons for wanting to stay healthy ourselves: It is much more important to preserve one's health over a long period of time than to frantically try and make healthy lifestyle changes out of fear when we suddenly turn fifty.

Is the answer to pop more and more vitamin pills? Vitamins, we know, are essential for growth, vitality, and healthy aging. But often overlooked is the importance of minerals; and trace minerals, in particular, are very difficult to get in the foods we eat. Unfortunately, much recent research indicates that most of these vitamin formulas, even if they do contain minerals, are assimilated in levels of only 10 percent or less. This is because they are artificially produced in a laboratory: The body simply regards it as another foreign substance. Many doctors believe, as we discussed in the last chapter, that isolated from the way in which they occur in nature, vitamins and minerals can even be toxic. They need to be in proper proportion. An excess can often lead to the same symptoms as a deficiency. And minerals need to be taken with enzymes to ensure proper absorption. In my opinion, and in the opinion of many experts working in the field today, the only solution to protect ourselves and our families is to find a whole food source that is still harvested in a natural mineral-rich environment, and to supplement our diets with plant-derived vitamins and minerals on a daily basis.

Examine the plethora of vitamin-mineral formulas on the shelves of drugstores today and you will hardly find two that are alike! This is because no one knows yet the proper proportions that the human body needs for optimum health and vitality. We know the minimum daily requirements—which we certainly are not getting from our foods—but only Mother Nature knows the secret harmonious balance of the perfect vitamin and mineral supplement.

After much research, I have come to the conclusion that whole foods and herbs provide the best source of energy necessary in assisting our bodies to maintain optimum health. Herbs, in their natural wholesome state, are a food, containing the vitamins, minerals, enzymes, and amino acids necessary, and in the correct proportions, to correct many of the malfunctions that plague our modern society. All great herbalists and natural healers believe in the vitalistic principal that the body, when given whole foods and herbal nutrition, has the inherent ability to self-correct.

The word "doctor" comes from the Latin word for "teacher." I have discovered, over the many years of experimenting with herbs, that I am my own best teacher. The body knows what it needs. I gave up going to traditional physicians years ago because philosophically the medical model is foreign to my consciousness and also because they have so seldom offered any relief! How many times have you heard of someone who went to a doctor for arthritis, chronic indigestion, or allergies (classic examples), only to return with a doomsday verdict that went something like this: "Well, here is a prescription that may help, but this is not really something we have a cure for. . . ." It happens every day: Doctors admit that they don't know the cause of most degenerative diseases and that there really isn't much that they can do about it.

What is horrific is that most prescriptions only exacerbate the problem by making the body dependent on an artificial chemical substance with side effects that are sometimes worse than the original symptomology. Drugs generally do not address the *cause* of disease; thus the condition continues to worsen, only it gets masked. We become addicted to our prescription fixes in the same way as an addict who must take a daily dose of heroin just to stay "normal." Witness the huge amount of antacids sold in this country.

The National Digestive Disease Information Clearing House in Bethesda, Maryland, published these statistics in the mid-1990s:

- There are 66 million reports of heartburn monthly.
- There are 20 million cases of gallstones.
- There are 20 million cases of irritable bowel.
- There are 22 million workdays lost to indigestion.[3]

These are the ones suffering from malnutrition the most, at least in our "well-fed," civilized world. And the antacid industry grows by leaps and bounds because the effect of eating them so regularly is to destroy the body's natural enzymes. Not only does the destruction of stomach acids cause dependency and make it difficult to absorb the nutrients from foods, they make it almost impossible for the body to break down fats. In addition, as we discussed earlier, antacids that contain aluminum are particularly dangerous for the bones and brain. And the newer forms—that used to be available by prescription only—interfere with proper liver functioning and hormone metabolism. Obviously these side effects can be a springboard for a host of other problems. This is just one example of how our addictions to drugs are killing us.

What is so remarkable is that there are natural solutions in the herbal kingdom that will come to our aid in so many ways. I am a woman in midlife and I have certainly had my share of preservatives, pesticide residues, hormone disrupters, chemical additives, and toxic metals in my food and from my environment. I have been a city dweller for the past fifteen years. As hard as I have tried to live organically, it is simply an inevitable fact that anyone alive today will be exposed to these toxins. I have had my share of ailments and symptoms from the classic degenerative diseases. But I have never had a physical complaint that herbs did not heal. I am truly astonished every time it happens.

There are potent herbs that will heal ulcers, arthritis, allergies, heart problems, digestive disorders, and many other degenerative disorders that doctors, for the most part, only know how to prescribe drugs for. Even if herbs cannot cure a serious degenerative disease, like some forms of arthritis, chronic fatigue, or a condition characterized by chronic pain, there are endless possibilities for successful treatment and pain management that are not harmful to the body the way that many drugs are, whether they be steroids, anti-depressants, aspirin, or anything else. (All drugs, even the drugstore variety, have serious side effects when ingested over a long period of time.)

Of course, we all fight an uphill battle with our daily dose of toxins we inevitably encounter, and many will die from cancer, heart disease, and diabetes, despite the most well-intentioned health regime. I remember how devastated I was when I learned that the pioneer Adelle Davis, author of numerous books on health and natural foods in the mid-1960s, died from cancer. However, even though we may become overwhelmed at the apocalyptic scenarios that we have created and their potential not only to undermine our personal health and vitality, but the future welfare of our children and the life of the entire planet, we must continue to strive for a more wholesome way of life. In my opinion, it is one of the most vital moral issues that we must urgently address if we are to move into the next millennium with pride and dignity.

It is through exploring, learning, and yes, careful experimentation, that we all become our own teachers. The remarkable thing about this kind of knowledge is that it continues to build, thus becoming a very stable structure, brick by brick. We learn from our past herbal legacy—which is certainly experiencing a new renaissance—and we learn from each other. We learn from the studies now being conducted on herbs and food supplements. And the more we learn, the more we begin to understand that one of the best ways of preserving health is by including phytonutrients in our diets for protection. In other words, we can use the phytochemicals that come from God's warehouse of herbs and whole foods not only to heal disease, but to help prevent it.

There are many reasons that one should think about preserving one's health by making dietary changes and adding supplements. There is a growing demand for pure, organic foods that are simply no longer available in today's normal grocery stores. Many hundreds of articles in major medical journals (such as the *New England Journal of Medicine,* the *Journal of the American Medical Association, Lancet,* the *British Medical Journal,* etc.) have produced study after study indicating that the less animal fat you eat, the healthier you will be and the longer your expected life span. There are studies on antioxidants and free radicals. There are studies on herbs and vitamins. There are studies on natural hormones from the plant kingdom. There are studies on the necessity of including phytonutrients in our daily diet.

The plant-based diet is experiencing a comeback. The National Cancer Institute and the Department of Health and Human Services now recommend five servings of fruits and vegetables a day. Unfortunately, almost 90 percent of Americans do not fulfill the daily requirements that satisfy their body's need for these whole foods. However, more and more people are realizing that to maintain optimum health we need to turn back to the herbal bounty Mother Nature has given us, for this bounty alone will supply what is lacking. Thus, phytonutrients are often packaged and sold in pill form.

Although this may not replace the benefits of whole foods, it can and should supplement diets that are not rich in raw foods, particularly fruits and vegetables.

Herbs & Formulas: Some Precautions

One of the greatest influences in my life has been Dr. John Christopher. I will discuss his healing philosophy more in the next chapter. It was from reading him that I discovered that the word "doctor" initially was derived from the word "teacher." He was a great herbalist and teacher and he left us a powerful legacy in his work. If you use herbal formulas, very likely you have tried one of Dr. Christopher's combinations. A major herb company, Nature's Way, had once distributed his formulas for over twenty years. His classic book, *The School of Natural Healing*, first published in 1976, has been reprinted eleven times and is still available. His simple motto, printed on the jacket cover, was, "God intended everyone to have the knowledge to properly take care of their own body."[4]

It is our responsibility to thus become more educated, and there are many books, tapes, schools, and herbal teachers today to help us grow in our herbal education. Herbs and herbal formulas are becoming more popular today in direct proportion to the growing demand Americans have to become informed consumers. We should rightfully beware of taking drugs, the effects of which we are largely ignorant, simply at the advice of a doctor. Likewise, one should beware of companies that tout "secret" herbal formulas. Herbal formulas should always be made known to the consumer. It is part of our herbal education.

The Dr. Christopher formulas, which I base my own formulas on, were never meant to be trade secrets, according to his son, David Christopher, because he did not want people to become dependent upon him.[5] All of his formulas were revealed in his book *The School of Natural Healing*, and can therefore be made by anyone. The herbs just need to be ground (or bought in powder form) and mixed. However, I would not advise an inexperienced person to randomly mix herbs with little or no knowledge of what they are doing. This can be potentially dangerous. Some herbs should not be taken together, and many herbs, with the exception of tonics, should not be taken continuously. (See "Frequently Asked Questions About Herbs" in chapter 1.)

However, there are some wonderful herb books available today that give recipes or formulas that are both safe and efficacious. I recommend, in addition to Dr. Christopher, the books by David Hoffman, Rosemary Gladstar, and Linda Rector Page for excellent formulas. (See bibliography.)

The Dr. Christopher formulas are available from his school in Utah, now operated by his son, David Christopher, and distributed by Christopher Enterprises. Although there are a couple of other companies that have distributed the Dr. Christopher formulas, some of them are not in their original form.

All phytonutrients are not safe just because they come from nature. Ma-huang is a case in point. Any weight-loss formula that contains ma-huang or ephedra (which Dr. Christopher did not use for weight loss) should have a label that contains a warning for those with diabetes, hypertension, or any kind of heart problem, and also a warning that the length of time it is taken should be short and monitored. Many distributors, especially in multilevel herbal marketing schemes, have to buy a certain amount of these products to keep their distributorship active. Thus, they are consuming large doses of herbs that they may not need, which certainly should not be used indefinitely on a daily basis, and which sometimes may cause distressing side effects. This is indiscriminate use of herbal products for a profit, a tendency that is becoming much too popular today.

At the time of this writing, the FDA has been investigating ma-huang-related deaths and will no doubt place severe restrictions on its use in the future. Yet, as we will see in the herbal section of this book, ma-huang (or ephedra) is a powerful and excellent herb for treating certain conditions other than weight loss. However, it is a common fad among many herb companies to use it for dieting. Present studies indicate it may not be safe to use (especially on a daily basis) with sedatives like Saint John's Wort. The current craze for herbal weight-loss products (especially if they are standardized, administered in high doses, or mixed with over-the-counter weight-loss products) is an area that needs much more research. In particular, stimulant and sedative herbs (ephedra and Saint John's Wort) do not make a good mix. It is becoming a favorite formula, popping up in numerous new companies, probably because many people wanting to lose weight tend to suffer depression while attempting to do so. In this case, it is best to examine the roots of the problem and not just treat the symptoms. Until one becomes an educated herbalist, herbal combinations and herb-drug combinations should be administered by a holistic health-care practitioner.

And there are other concerns about some of the herbal weight-loss products that are popular today. A dangerous trend I have noticed in a couple of companies is the addition of DHEA, or other hormones. Why? This robs a person of the choice about whether to take hormones when they take a weight-loss product, the contents of which they may be largely unaware of. It is very premature to access what the implications of this could be, but I think it is dangerous to take hormones without testing blood levels for the need for hormones: DHEA, like estrogen, is implicated in cancers of the reproductive tract in both sexes, especially in large doses.

Another area of alarming research right now is the massive self-administration of weight-loss products with foods that contain exicotoxins. These chemicals and food additives, especially monosodium glutamate, aspartame, and other artificial sweeteners, have been strongly implicated with brain and behavior disorders, especially ADD (attention deficit disorder), dementia, and Alzheimer's disease.[6] As Dr. Russell Blaylock pointed out in his book *Excitotoxins*, a typical weight-loss diet consists largely of diet phosphates (soft drinks) and many foods that contain artificial sweeteners. Individuals using this diet may be at particular risk for developing brain diseases as they age, since consistent use of such harmful chemicals can severely damage neural pathways to the brain. Herbal weight-loss products, if they contain ma-huang, or over-the-counter products that curb appetite can also tend to make a person feel hyper, adding even more to a potential growing mental and physical disorder. In addition, any product that curbs the appetite lessens the probability that one will eat three balanced meals a day, and increases the tendency to consume these other, more dangerous foods.

In a conversation I had with David Christopher, he said, "Dr. Christopher is pure in the sense of Hippocrates: that is, the body heals itself if given the right environment."[7] This environment, first and foremost, consists in whole foods the way that Mother Nature made them, not in the present form in which so many modern foods appear on supermarket shelves, laden with chemicals and preservatives. When the body is properly cleansed and nourished, it has a tendency to repair itself. It will never have this opportunity when bombarded with poor foods, chemical additives, and environmental pollutants on a regular basis. Too many modern doctors often evade the real issue by telling the patient that he or she has a chronic disease—which frequently affects the body parts actively attempting to cleanse the body of its poisons: The liver, kidneys, skin, bowel, and digestive tract.

David Christopher also feels that, in attempting to create rigid methods of standardization, many modern herbalists, wanting to win the acceptance of the medical community, are moving more and more toward the allopathic model (or the traditional medical model), in the delusion that it is more efficacious if a herb is administered in higher doses. Many holistic practitioners, on the other hand, feel that a huge dose of an herb may not be more beneficial. More may not be better! The whole tradition of homeopathic medicine has given us a legacy that indicates, in fact, that less may be better, if delivered in a holistic way.

We will discuss the pros and cons of standardized herbs in the next chapter. I want to stress that my own personal preference, however, is to take herbs in the form in which Mother Nature made them whenever possible. In isolating components from the plant kingdom and selling them as over-the-counter supplements, we run the risk of side effects. In many cases, much more research needs to be done on what these repercussions are. For example, we now know that one of the flavonoids, Quercetin (a popular supplement sold in many health food stores), is potentially carcinogenic.[9]

Another herb that has stirred up a lot of controversy is licorice. However, in this case, the dangers may have been overstated. Licorice, especially in combination with other herbs, can be effective in treating acid indigestion. Many herbal compounds that are alternative antacids contain licorice. Licorice has, as one of its main ingredients, glycyrrhizic acid (GLA), which has been found to raise blood pressure in some people. So another synthesized form of licorice was made that has 95 percent of this component removed, and it works to suppress stomach acid but not to cure the long-term causes of this problem. (Traditionally, one of the uses of licorice has been used to treat gastritis and ulcers.) When this constituent is removed, you do not get the full beneficial effects of the whole herb, which also acts as an anti-inflammatory and blood-sugar balancer. In addition, in women, it is an excellent source of natural, safe estrogen.

Numerous holistic doctors advise taking DGL, or the deglycyrrhizinated form of licorice; but most herbalists I know would advise against it, and the reason is simple: The kind God made just might be better for curing the disease (i.e., healing the mucous membranes), not just the targeted short-term effects (neutralizing stomach acid). If using the whole herb does cause an elevation in blood pressure (which should always be monitored when adding anything new to the diet), then one can switch to something else. In the herbal kingdom, there are many possibilities. (See the chart on digestion, page 322.)

One modern herbalist has noted that "the toxicity of licorice has been greatly exaggerated by well-meaning quasi-herbalists and media types."[9] The reason, by the way, that licorice is not as dangerous as ma-huang in raising blood pressure is that licorice has adaptogenic or tonic characteristics (which means it has more of a homeostatic effect) and ma-huang does not.

As a precautionary note, here are some other things an informed consumer should know about herbs:

- Choose herbs that are organically grown. The vast majority, even in health food stores, are not. Read labels as you do when you buy food. Herbs are very concentrated foods. This is what part of their essence is: They are the distilled, concentrated life energy of the plant. Therefore, if you are consistently eating herbs laced with pesticides or additives, you are diligently feeding a concentrated dose of poison into your body.

- Buy herbs fresh. The advantage of pills is that they are easy to take and are relatively inexpensive. But the shelf life of most herbs in capsules or tablets is less than a year. People who complain that the herbs they tried did not work are probably experiencing lack of results for one of two reasons: The herbs were not taken long enough, or they were so old as to be of practically no value. Absorption of the active ingredients is not as efficient in pill form as when the herb is taken in an infusion (tea) or extract. Herbs stay fresher much longer when they are dried and roughly cut. Powdering herbs creates an opportunity for oxygen and moisture to more quickly break down the vital active constituents.

- If an herb is causing you a lot of grief, *stop taking it.* Minor unwanted side effects, such as headache, nausea, or loose bowel, should be distinguished, however, from more serious ones such as increased blood pressure, heart palpitations, or mental disorientation. Some side effects result from the cleansing action of the herb, a topic we will explore more in the next section.

- Do not take medicinal herbs for an extended period of time, unless the herbs are primarily tonics (of which there are many). Adaptogens and antioxidants generally fall into this category and can be taken indefinitely, although it is good to take a break occasionally. Nourishing herbs are whole foods that can be taken as preventive supplements. But do not take any herb that stimulates or sedates indefinitely. If you are taking herbs to treat a chronic condition, rotate the herbs. There are many to choose from. Anti-inflammatories are generally safe to take over a long period of time if rotated. Some immunostimulants or immunomodulators are safe if taken over long periods of time to rebuild the immune system. See the charts in part 3 for a quick reference to these categories of herbs.

+ Ask the manufacturer of the herbs you are taking:

> Where the herb comes from,
>
> How it is processed (if fillers are added, if heat is used in drying, if the herb is fractionated), and
>
> What exactly is in the capsule or extract you are buying, including percentages of the herb or herbs.

If the supplier can't answer these questions or hedges in their response, go someplace else.

The increased interest in using phytonutrients to supplement diet, to heal disorders, and to offer protection from the environment has stirred up a heated debate among doctors and herbalists about how these supplements should be administered. Standardization is at the heart of this debate. We will examine it in the next chapter, along with a brief sketch of the three herbalists who have most influenced me in my own herbal philosophy.

Notes

1. P. Tompkins and C. Bird, *Secrets of the Soil* (New York: Harper & Row, 1989), p. xx.
2. J. Loggie, "Hypertension in the pediatric patient," *Journal of Pediatrics* 94 (1979): 685.
3. Informational brochure, National Digestive Disease Information Clearing House, Box NDDIC, 900 Rockville Pike, Bethesda, Maryland, 20892.
4. J. R. Christopher, *The School of Natural Healing* (Springville, Utah: Christopher Publications, 1991).

5. David Christopher, personal phone conversation, 10 February 1998.

6. R. Blaylock, *Excitotoxins, the Taste That Kills* (Sante Fe: Health Press, 1996).

7. David Christopher conversation.

8. Ibid.

9. See, for example, J. T. MacGregor and L. Jurd, *Mutat. Res.* 54 (1978): 297–309; E. Middleton, *Biochem. Pharmacol.* 31 (1982), 1449–1453. In: Herb Research Foundation Information packet, TIPS, August 1984.

10. D. Mowrey, *Herbal Tonic Therapies* (New York: Wings Books, 1993), p. 325.

In a grasping world, herbs are always giving. They show us how health care ought to be: conscious of the whole person.

—LINDA RECTOR PAGE, AUTHOR,
"THE HERBAL PHARMACIST"

5

Herbal versus Medical Approaches to Healthy Living

John Raymond Christopher, John Lust, and Rosemary Gladstar have all contributed greatly to the growing body of herbal knowledge in this century and I gratefully build on the heritage that has gone before me. Let's examine how the herbal tradition distinguishes the work of these great teachers (another word for "doctor," remember!) from the current medical model as I understand it.

The Christopher School of Natural Healing

Many herbs are medicinal, but the purpose of a holistic health regime is not just to treat symptoms. That is the traditional medical model, and it sometimes has its uses, especially for treating emergencies. However, in the philosophy of Dr. Christopher, we need an approach by which a person may attack the cause, not just the effects, of illness. In order to understand treatment and health maintenance using the Dr. Christopher method, we first need to understand the difference between the two approaches to medicine. They are the vitalist and the atomistic approaches, and they are diametrically opposed.

In the vitalist point of view, the body is always attempting to move toward wholeness, toward wellness. The vitalist tries to work with the body through herbs and whole foods, with the philosophical belief that when the body is properly nourished, it heals itself. Herbal treatments therefore enable you to activate your own resources to combat disease and build the immune system. There are literally thousands of herbal books and magazines available today targeted for anyone from the beginner to the most sophisticated herbal pharmacist. Like Dr. Christopher said, we must learn to become our own teachers. In this alternative tradition, the herbal way enables us to take charge of our own lives, health, and well-being, not only on the physical but also the mental and spiritual levels.

The atomistic philosophy believes that the body is composed of atoms; that is, we are only matter, and the consciousness we possess is only connected to brain tissue. In this model, the body must continually have its symptoms treated, because the body does not know how to heal itself. This is a reductionistic approach: Everything is understood by breaking it down into parts. This is vastly different from the philosophy that believes the whole is greater than the sum of its parts.

The atomistic approach is to block or stop a bodily function, for example, a cough. An atomistic approach is that a cough is bad, therefore make it go away as quickly as possible by suppressing it as completely as possible. A vitalistic approach is to take herbs that will work with the body, and in most cases, make you cough more! Coughing seeks to loosen phlegm, and so the vitalistic approach is to administer an expectorant. This is working with the body to self-correct. This approach enables one to mobilize the body's own natural defenses to stay healthy. Many times, when we treat cold symptoms with drugs, it only serves to drag out the cold. When we treat it herbally, it often hastens the healing process.

Dr. Jensen, author of *Empty Harvest*, explains how this works: "Just what [are] the effects of stopping the elimination of all the cell waste thrown off by cold symptoms? If you stop a cold, you stop what the body is accomplishing by the action of a cold."[1]

The first step in ridding the body of disease in the Christopher holistic model is to find and eliminate the cause. The cause may be a poisoned emotion or a poisoned environmental toxin. It may be the kind of food that is continually being ingested or the uninterrupted stress one is subjected to on a daily basis. Dr. Christopher believed diet was very often the cause, but that all factors should be investigated. Symptoms are only expressions of the body's attempt to heal itself. They are not the cause of disease. Therefore, holistic healers and alternative physicians direct specific treatment to root causes whenever possible. Herbs in particular are effective in doing this. Dr. Christopher believed that most major illnesses can be cured by a limited fast and cleansing herbs, along with the elimination of toxic foods when the diet is resumed, particularly those that are mucous forming.

One of the things Dr. Christopher said was:

> As your body begins to cleanse, you will probably experience periodic aches and pains in the areas where the cleansing is most acute. Where waste is loading the elimination system, there may be times when you are feeling very, very rough! Do not panic . . . be comforted that the healing process is well underway, and the sooner such discomforts come, the better, for this means that the toxins and poisons are being eliminated.[2]

There are four major elimination organs through which the body first attempts to cleanse itself: the bowel, the kidney, the lungs, and the skin. Different people experience the elimination of toxicity in different ways when first starting on a herbal program, or one high in phytonutrients, such as wheat grass, algae, or vegetable juices. Some will experience an increase in gastrointestinal distress. Others may have more mucus congestion. Still others will experience skin eruptions. Normally, the skin, bowel, and lungs are the first line of defense against toxins. If the intestines are overburdened with excessive stress from a poor diet, the burden is transferred to the liver, which is often the last line of defense the body has. When a deficient liver is ineffective in defending the body, excess toxins are dumped into the blood and from there go to the glands, tissues, or organs that are the weakest part of the body. Hence, cleansing is vital to protect one from disease. Dr. Christopher was famous for his excellent cleansing formulas. Cleansing herbs are not necessarily laxative, which should not be taken over an extended period of time. Many cleansing herbs are just nutrients that initially attempt to detoxify the body, and some, like milk thistle or seaweed greens, can be taken indefinitely without disturbing side effects. Here are some examples of cleansing or detoxifying herbs that work on different body systems:

Bowel: aloe, cascara sagrada, senna, psyllium

Mucus: lobelia, comfrey, cayenne, yarrow

Blood: dandelion, burdock, milk thistle, algae, goldenseal

Diuretics: juniper, buchu, uva ursi

General (may affect several systems at once): licorice, chaparral, sarsaparilla, red clover, Pau d' Arco, cat's claw

Check the herbal section of this book for specifics on each herb.

Detoxifying generally includes a lot of vegetable juices and olive oil, combined with a fast from solid food. Some herbs that are blood purifiers or alternatives are also rebuilding/nourishing herbs, e.g., burdock, algae, and dandelion.

As the body is cleansed, it needs to be rebuilt and properly nourished. Dr. Christopher believed that when cleansed and nourished with the correct herbal nutrients, the body will go to work immediately to rectify whatever might be wrong with it. To rebuild our immune systems and maintain good health, according to the Christopher model, we must return to whole foods, preferably grown organically. Packaged, frozen, canned, and chemical-laden foods are dead. Food grown on organic, nutrient-rich soil is vital to optimum health. If we transfer all of the responsibility for the production of our food to faceless growers who unwittingly buy devitalized fertilizer laced with toxic waste, we set ourselves up for abuse.

In the Christopher philosophy, one must include plenty of foods that are rich in enzymes, which are the life force of the plant kingdom. In his mucous-free diet theory, lifeless foods cause mucous, congestion, and toxins. Dr. Christopher had an astonishing rate of healing people whom doctors had turned away as hopeless. However, it is a sad fact that people too often lose hope because they continue to be treated by those whose success rate is rare, at best, at least in terms of the major degenerative diseases. An on-line report I recently read quoted Dr. Hardin Jones, who said, "My studies have proven that untreated cancer victims actually live up to four times longer than treated individuals."[3] According to Edward Griffin, author of *World Without Cancer*, the average cure rate for cancer by medical doctors is 17 percent, excluding skin cancers.[4] Chemotherapy-treated patients fare even worse. Dr. John Cairns, of the Harvard University School of Public Health, has said that he believes that only 2 to 3 percent of cancer victims are treated successfully with chemotherapy.[5] However, it is unlawful for anyone to "treat" cancer unless he or she is a physician. The reason herbalists must legally abstain from making claims is to avoid offending the American Medical Association. Dr. Christopher was arrested five times on charges of "practicing medicine" without a license. Yet he had a phenomenal success in treating patients who had found no relief from conventional doctors. Although persecuted by orthodox medicine for his practice and beliefs, he was undaunted in his concern for suffering people, and at the same time he maintained a keen sense of humor in the face of great difficulties and enormous attorney bills.

Most of today's herbalists do not have to fight the battles Dr. Christopher did. He is considered by many to be the pioneer of today's modern herbal renaissance. Before he became a certified Herbal Pharmacist, he suffered from rheumatoid arthritis (and was confined to a wheelchair), stomach ulcers, and cancer. He cured himself of all of his illnesses and went on to cure countless others. He was inspired to become a herbalist when, from his wheelchair, he picked up the Bible one day to the passage in Ezekiel 47, which reads, "And the fruit of the tree shall be for meat, and the leaf thereof for medicine." His ability to heal people with his famous Dr. Christopher formulas gained him such notoriety that, before he was forced to shut down his practice, he was seeing eighty to ninety patients a day. At that time, Utah legislation did not permit him to practice as a herbalist and a naturopathic doctor. He remained committed to his mission of healing, however. After being forced to abandon his work, he went on the lecture circuit, traveling internationally and visiting 50–100 cities each year. He was normally booked a year in advance.

One of his great contributions in the herbal tradition was the exploration of the breakdown of the mineral content of herbs. His studies at various herbal institutes led him to an understanding of the more technical aspects of herbs, which were relatively unknown to earlier herbalists, such as Jethro Kloss. He believed that herbs were the most perfect food and offered a complete array of minerals in their safest, most available form. The reason he advised against many mineral supplements available today is simple: Assimilation. He once said:

> [W]e can get a shovelful of the dust of the earth and . . . pharmaceutically grind it down to a point of medicinal fineness and put it into capsules and take it. All right, we're getting these minerals: the iron, sulphur, magnesium . . . They are accepted into the body and accepted very easily, but not much of it is assimilated. The essential thing is that each herb that grows on the face of this earth has its own way of demanding the minerals that it needs. For example, garlic demands sulfur . . . The sulfur minerals that are in the earth can be beneficial, but they leave side effects, whereas the sulfur that has accumulated in the garlic is beneficial with no side effects and no after effects. It is already assimilated, so it is acceptable to the body.[6]

Dr. Christopher advocated using the whole herb as a tea whenever possible, because it was the fastest, surest way for the herb to gain access to the body. He felt that even in tincture form certain particles in the herb were lost. This is in marked distinction to many modern herbalists who advise tinctures, extracts, and standardized capsules for maximum potency. However, Dr. Christopher always preferred to think of herbs—even cleansing herbs—as foods, and believed in using them in their most natural form possible.

He organized the School for Natural Healing in 1953, where he taught the many ways herbs are grown, harvested, compounded, and used in various treatments. He taught his students as simply as he taught his patients, with a parting admonition that this was a do-it-yourself kit. The School even today employs Dr. Christopher's "keep it simple" philosophy but uses modern technology to deliver an unprecedented home study curriculum. It is now directed by his son, David Christopher. Today, thousands safely apply the Christopher methodology thanks to his directorship.[7]

Dr. Christopher is perhaps most famous for his combinations, or formulas, some of which came through experimentation, and some of which just came to him from the "universal mind." He said in one of his lectures that these particular formulas came in a "flash," very quickly, and all he did was write them down. He lectured practically nonstop until his death. In one of his final lectures, he said, "The Lord was kind enough to show me the way and I just want to show the way to others."[8]

John Lust: Bridging the Gap Between the Old Traditions and Modern Phytomedicine

John Lust is another famous herbalist, teacher, and writer who carried on a family tradition begun in the early part of this century. His uncle, Dr. Benedict Lust, is known as the father of naturopathy. He was born into an environment where herbal healing and organic living were natural concepts, although his uncle, like Dr. Christopher, had to fight an uphill battle with the medical establishment. Benedict Lust, along with John's father, opened up the first health-food store in New York in 1896 and, shortly thereafter, two sanatoriums. John's uncle Benedict had learned much from a priest-physician by the name of Father Kneipp in Germany, who had cured him of consumption. Doctors had told him he would probably die, since his disease was too far progressed for the medical cures of the period. After experiencing a complete recovery with Fr. Kneipp's herbs and water cure, his life mission was devoted to helping others in America.

John's legacy in continuing this mission was in education. After working in the family store and sanatoriums and keeping extensive records, he published his famous *The Herb Book*, which he considered to be a synthesis of two generations of information. It is one of the most comprehensive herbals ever published, with hundreds of categories, cataloged by plant, symptom, and botanical name. It includes herbal legend, history, harvesting and storing herbs, how to make herbal preparations, glossaries of medicinal effects and botanical terms, a compendium of botanical medicine, and sections on spices, herbal cosmetics, and vitamins and minerals. It has been a constant reference source for me for over twenty years.

John worked at his uncle's American School of Naturopathy, which eventually granted degrees in this healing art, and published many small books on herbs because he felt that the educational approach was the most efficacious way to reach large numbers of people. In his words,

> [N]aturopathy relies on simple herbal remedies—in conjunction with fasting, exercise, fresh air, sunshine, water and diet—to help the body regain health naturally . . . [The] basic assumption behind natural healing is that man is part of a continuum of being. Since he is a living being, his physical and mental condition is linked especially to the properties and influences of natural organic substances.[9]

He felt that naturopathy continued to survive, despite great opposition, because it offered something that modern treatments lacked, that is, "treatments which worked in harmony with life and weren't antagonistic to it."[10] At the same time, he showed hopeful concern that herbalism could coexist successfully with Western medicine and he witnessed many scientific breakthroughs with plants, which he saw as a positive development. He acknowledged that *The Herb Book* had led to many modern investigations.[11]

And indeed, such has been the case, as modern researchers continue to take an ever-increasing interest in the medicinal properties of plants. Although standardization of herbs was not popular during the period when John Lust wrote his classic book, it is now a major debate in the herbal community. Before moving on, I would like to explain how the process of standardizing herbs evolved. For the greater part of this century, American pharmaceutical companies took no interest in medicinal herbs because plants cannot be patented. They were, however, interested in isolating the "active" constituents of some plants for specific purposes, such as the cardiac stimulant, digitalis, from foxglove, or aspirin from the salicylate in white willow. What continues to confound researchers, however, is that frequently the isolated constituent is less effective than the crude herb, or it has different effects.

Extracts from the whole herb—or crude extracts—that have no monetary value to the pharmaceutical companies consistently seem to have greater therapeutic value. Toxicity is also less likely to occur when using the whole herb, or in a crude extract, than in using isolated active constituents. Nonetheless, the potency of herbal extracts is always difficult to determine because the herbal strength varies with the soil, growing conditions, harvesting, storage, and a variety of other factors. One batch of any given herb might have a lower level of biologically active constituents than another, and this can pose problems for health-care practitioners inclined to use herbs as an adjunct to their therapies.

As the interest in using pharmaceutical agents from plants developed, so did the insistence on quality control and accepted standardized levels to insure adequate dosages. This also allows for controlled studies to be performed measuring an herb's efficacy. Proponents of standardization say we can reliably count on receiving the same quantity of the active biological ingredients per unit taken, and thus the consumer can rely on a specific quantity of these constituents to be present in the herb when she or he buys it.

Standardization has become popular in Europe, where nearly all doctors and pharmacists study and know herbal therapy and incorporate it into their practice. However, the regulation of herbs in Europe clashes with the way they are regulated in the United States, since there phytomedicines are generally considered drugs rather than "dietary supplements" like they are in America. This is why the bulk of clinical trials on phytomedicines have been done in Europe. There are many herbalists in the United States who are fighting to keep herbs classified as "food" and not a "drug" for several reasons, as pointed out by Robert McCaleb, the president of the Herb Research Foundation:

> [D]ietary supplement legislation in the United States has been designed to provide the public with access to scientific information about the uses of botanicals and other natural products without requiring an unachievable standard of evidence, such as the one applied in the U.S. for the approval of new drugs. . . . [M]any botanicals are used in the same way as nutrients to maintain healthy body functioning . . . a rigid drug regulatory system ignores the multi-cultural nature of botanical medicine and undervalues the knowledge gained from historical use of these remedies . . . While high-tech phytomedicines may be the wave of the future . . . much of the world will continue to use low-tech formulations, just as they have for generations.[12]

Some herbalists are concerned that standardization separates herbal constituents so much that it makes them too much like drugs, with the inevitable side effects. One can use the salicylate from white willow, for instance, without the risk of intestinal upset or bleeding, which is a known negative effect of aspirin. The actions of herbs tend to be more supportive of the body's normal functions and frequently an herb is multi-effective in its actions. Isolated components, or phytomedicines that are more drug-like, tend to be suppressive of normal functions, since they are more targeted for specific effects. As one modern herbalist, who is completely opposed to standardization, says:

> As naturally concentrated foods, herbs have the unique ability to address a multiplicity of problems simultaneously. In most cases, the full medicinal value of herbs is in their internal complexity . . . [M]any of the constituents within a whole herb are unknown— even to modern science—and internal chemical reactions within and among herbs are even less understood . . . the result [of standardization] is an overly refined product . . . It's a case of government regulation and orthodox medicine trying to make herbal healing fit into a laboratory drug mold.[13]

My own feelings about standardization lie somewhere between the two extremes. On the one hand, I think it is a positive move that the mainstream American consciousness is moving closer to accepting herbal remedies and part of the reason lies in the fact that we now have quantitative data, based on objective studies, to replace old superstitions about herbs based primarily on subjective impressions. Some of the newer plant species being discovered in jungles like South America, for instance, have been studied extensively and now show positive potential for future use as cancer and arthritis remedies. Other herbal constituents, of which we were largely unaware until this generation, hold remarkable hope for newly emerging diseases like AIDS and chronic fatigue syndrome. Some of this exciting research has been included in this herbal, along with the more traditional applications for which the herb has been used in the past.

Some plants, like Saint John's Wort, have never been tested for targeted effects (e.g., depression) except in standardized doses. Therefore, we still don't know if lower doses, or dosages that do not include the recommended "Guaranteed Potency," will have the same effects in clinical settings. This is where each of us, as our own herbal teacher, must experiment and decide for ourselves. (For more on this herb, see chapter 7.)

I think standardization is safest when the herbal extracts are made only from plants that have been subjected to quality control measurements and when the active constituents are returned to the whole plant in the final product, thus insuring the inherent system of checks and balances ordained by Mother Nature. Otherwise, we run the risk of creating an imbalanced drug-like effect, and the synergistic actions possible for the herb are lost. I also think it is vital to use herbs as nutrients to encourage overall body balancing. Thus, it is imperative that we keep herbs listed as food supplements so we have the choice to use them as preventative tonics as well as for the treatment of illnesses.

John Lust, who stood on the threshold of traditional herbalism and its more modern applications, summed up our present dilemma when he wrote:

[F]rom the vantage point of the late twentieth century, we have both the perspective and the resources to assess the true relationship—physical and psychological—of plants to man, to test for ourselves what remains valid today of the ancient claims and beliefs.[14]

Rosemary Gladstar and the Modern Herbal Renaissance

In the 1960s, a young woman named Rosemary Gladstar dropped out of college and moved to the Washington coastal wilderness to follow her dream of living close to nature. She studied the herbal wisdom of the elders she found there. A few years later, she bought a horse and, taking no food, foraged off the land along the Pacific Coast Trail for four months—with her two-year-old son.

The woman often called the "Godmother of the Herbal Renaissance," when asked how she became an herbalist, once replied, "All I knew was that I loved plants, loved what my grandmother taught me, and gravitated to the people who loved herbs as I did."[15] This simplicity and humility, paired with an amazing charisma, dominates the style of Rosemary, one of the most powerful woman healers of our time. Mark Blumenthal, the director of the American Botanical Council, once summed up her achievements by stating:

> Rosemary is a fountain of medicinal herb knowledge . . . But what makes her so special is that she's also a charismatic organizer. Rosemary creates herbal institutions. If she isn't the Godmother of Herbalism today, I don't know who is.[16]

Like Dr. Christopher and John Lust, who were so instrumental in shifting the herbal consciousness of an earlier era, Rosemary Gladstar is becoming a legend in her own lifetime. A list of her achievements should indicate why.

In 1972, she opened up a small herb shop in Sebastopol, California, called Rosemary's Garden. She expanded the herbal consciousness of the locality by inviting such visionaries as Dr. Christopher, Marcia Starck, and Anne Wigmore. At the same time, she began making herbal tea blends for her friends and immediate community that later became known as Traditional Medicinals, one of the nation's leading herbal medicine tea companies.

She soon was off to greener pastures, however, leaving the former businesses in other competent hands. In 1982, she founded the California School of Herbal Studies. The school started "very organically," explains Rosemary. At first, it was only a series of workshops she developed. However, "people wanted more information. They were hungry . . . I too shared the same hunger and desire for greater understanding."[17] A friend offered to house the school on an eighty-acre ranch in an idyllic little place called Emerald Valley, in Forestville, California. You will never forget Emerald Valley if you ever get a chance to visit it; it is a mecca of nature's bounty, and currently attracts students from a wide variety of backgrounds. Today it still offers one of the nation's most respected courses in medical herbology.

Once the school was running smoothly, Rosemary organized an herb gathering at a hot springs resort in Breitenbush, Oregon's Cascade Mountains, and shortly afterward, in 1986, moved to Vermont, where she opened up Sage Mountain Herbal Retreat Center and Botanical Sanctuary. Breitenbush has continued to be an annual event, attracting famous herbalists worldwide. At Sage Mountain, she helped her stepdaughters start a business called Sage Mountain Herbal Products, while she devoted her energies to developing one of New England's foremost learning centers for herbs and earth awareness.

Rosemary has a relationship with her plants that is very familial. Describing her favorite herbs, she uses phrases that remind one of relationships with people: "I have a love affair with echinacea"; "Skullcap is a friendly plant"; "I admire dandelion for its tenacity . . . [I]t is a warrior plant"; "I consider garlic part of my family."[18]

In 1993, she published *Herbal Healing for Women*, which sold over 100,000 copies and is still in print. It is an excellent herbal remedy book, and additionally it is filled with rich insights about women's developmental cycles. Since I also wrote a book exploring both the psychological and physical dimensions of the woman's aging process.[19] I find much to honor in Rosemary's understanding of core issues vital to a woman's soul. Like so many of us, when Rosemary entered menopause, she found support and safety in a circle of women friends. But what was unique to Rosemary's style is that she organized workshops and conferences wherever she went to create a forum where women could have the opportunity to share their anxieties about the aging process, as well as learn herbal therapies targeted specifically for older women's needs. In Rosemary's opinion, aging is an opportunity for unprecedented growth; "You've got to grow old before you become wise."[20]

In 1990, she hosted the first International Herb Symposium, creating a forum for herbalists worldwide to network. Her concern at the time was that medical herbalism was replacing traditional earth-centered practices. "When traditional herbalism clashes with science, I go with tradition," she says.[21] A principle reason is that standardization often produces conflicting results from the traditional use of the whole plant. Concerned about the bad press over comfrey, Rosemary wrote, "[J]udging a plant's action of the basis of a single chemical component is like judging a person's character on the basis of a single personality trait."[22] In other words, isolating specific components of a plant, like pharmacists do for drug manufacturing or, in some cases, standardization, can also cause certain chemicals of that specific plant to become quite dangerous.

She is also concerned about the current tension between the two traditions. "The scientists condescend the traditional herbalists. And the traditional herbalists feel intimidated by the scientists and resentful of them."[23] This tension is heightened by the controversy over licensing, which disturbs Rosemary because "it takes herbalism away from the people, away from its natural roots. Standards are fine in theory, but in real life, they always become political and bureaucratic . . . [N]o license guarantees quality. The answer is to teach the public about healing so they recognize quality care and knows who's good."[24] Asked how one is to recognize a good herbalist, Rosemary replied,

> The same way you recognize good doctors—by who they are, what they know, and their reputations. Look for herbalists you feel are

honest, have integrity, and inspire your trust. Ask how long they've been working with herbs.[25]

It was around 1992 that Rosemary began noticing that plants were becoming less available in their native habitats. She became so concerned that she decided ("through a message I heard directly from the heart of the earth")[26] to start a nonprofit organization called United Plant Savers. Its aim was the preservation of Native American medicinal plants. In 1994, the Fourth International Herb Symposium was held as a benefit for the budding vision, and in recent years botanical sanctuaries have sprung up in partnership with United Plant Savers in numerous parts of the country. Many herbalists today try to follow the path of ecological wildcrafting, and the reason is simple. As market competition and profits rise, conservationists fear the current herbal craze could mean the extinction of some of our most valued herbal plants. As many as 250 wild medicinal herbs may now be threatened. These herbalists involved with United Plant Savers advocate not only eco-harvesting of wild plants, but also cultivation of endangered varieties. One of the major distributors of bulk herbs in the United States, Frontier, is a staunch supporter of Rosemary's hope of saving endangered plants and has begun to grow threatened herbs, like goldenseal, in protected habitats. In 1994, she began formulating herbal formulas for Frontier, which now distributes them worldwide.

Rosemary's initial dream—the little herb shop in Sebastopol that she started twenty years earlier—has certainly borne good fruit.

Asked what the secret of her success is, she once answered, "The seed of my success in the business realm is really the same seed that allows me to live and breathe and be a part of this great earth."[27] And although all of her endeavors have turned out to be enormously successful, she often has left them in the hands of someone else, "who can do the job better," while she sought a quiet place in the garden to meditate and "to travel deep."[28]

Perhaps it is her detachment and humility that are the characteristics I admire most about Rosemary. She never strove for success, only to share what she knew. "I consider myself successful at something if it takes me one step closer to understanding."[29] Rosemary believes she still has much to learn from plants and this, in itself, is very humbling. "I believe very deeply that humility if necessary to be a good healer."[30] The major intent in all of her organizing has always been balance: to use what is available "for the good of all of our relationships. . . . ask the nature spirits how this fits into their divine plan".[31]

It has not always been easy. Each endeavor has been a risk. However, if risks are frightening, Rosemary says it signifies that one needs to stretch:

> Whether it's your business that needs to grow and stretch or yourself, you usually reach a place of fright. And you'll have to risk to step through. To be creative in a business world means risking, stepping beyond what seems possible.[32]

Rosemary's phenomenal success as an herbalist and teacher can be summed up on a simple note of gratitude: "[I] just feel very privileged to have been able to live a life I love."[33]

All of these herbal teachers have helped many thousands of people reconnect with the powerful healing potential of little weeds that often grow in our own backyards.

In reclaiming our connection to the greening power of nature— what St. Hildegard of Bingen called "veriditas"—we are discovering anew the true connection of the life force within all of creation. This is the journey that reconnects us with one another, as we rediscover the blessings placed here for our mutual assistance by our Creator. As another of my favorite herbal teachers, Linda Rector Page (author of *The Herbal Pharmacist*), so eloquently put it, "The only way to see the incredible power of God is to undertake something so great that you cannot do it alone."[34]

Notes

1. B. Jensen and M. Anderson, *Empty Harvest: Understanding the Link Between Our Food, Our Immunity, and Our Planet* (Garden City Park, NY: Avery Publishing Group, 1990), p. 105.

2. J. Christopher, *The School of Natural Healing* (Springville, Utah: Christopher Publications, 20th edition, 1996), p. 570.

3. On-line report, H. Jones, "A report on cancer: speech delivered to the American Cancer Society's 11th Annual Science Writer's Conference," New Orleans, LA, published in *The Choice,* May 1977.

4. E. Griffin, *World Without Cancer* (American Media Publishers, 1997).

5. Ibid. See also J. Cairns, "The treatment of disease and the war against cancer," *Scientific American* (November 1985).

6. Quoted in R. Conrow and A. Hecksel, *Herbal Pathfinders* (Santa Barbara: Woodbridge Press, 1983), p. 236.

7. For further information on the School, please contact The School of Natural Healing, 25 West 200 South, Springville, Utah, 84663.

8. Conrow, *Herbal Pathfinders*, p. 238.

9. J. Lust, *The Herb Book* (New York: Bantam Books, 1974), p. 7.

10. Ibid.

11. Conrow, *Herbal Pathfinders*, p. 117.

12. R. McCaleb, *Herb Research News* 2, no. 2 (1997): 3.

13. L. R. Page, *The Herbal Pharmacist* (1991). Published by the author.

14. Lust, *The Herb Book*, p. 9.

15. M. Castleman, "Rosemary Gladstar: The Godmother of the Herbal Renaissance," *Vegetarian Times* (August 1991): 66.

16. Ibid.

17. S. Maine, *Creating an Herbal Business.*

18. Unpublished interview with Rosemary Gladstar.

19. M. Compton, *Women at the Change* (Llewellyn Publications, 1998).

20. M. Castleman, "Rosemary Gladstar: The Godmother of the Herbal Renaissance," *Vegetarian Times* (August 1991): 69.

21. Ibid., p. 68.

22. R. Gladstar, *Herbal Healing for Women* (New York: Simon & Schuster, 1993), p. 238.

23. Castleman, p. 68.

24. Ibid., p. 69.

25. Unpublished interview with Rosemary Gladstar.

26. S. Maine, *Creating an Herbal Business.*

27. Ibid.

28. Ibid.

29. Ibid.

30. Castleman, p. 70.

31. Maine.

32. Ibid.

33. Unpublished interview with Rosemary Gladstar.

34. L. R. Page, *The Herbal Pharmacist*, p. 16.

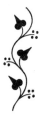

When we talk about health care reform, we [should] put preventive nutrition very high on the list, and that would include antioxidant supplementation.

—ADRIANNE BENDICH, CLINICAL RESEARCH
SCIENTIST AT HOFFMAN–LA ROCHE

6

Free Radicals
and Inexpensive
Lifesavers

As more and more people fear that the war on cancer is being lost, that our food supply is being irrevocably poisoned, that deadly "superbacteria" that are antibiotic resistant are evolving, there is simultaneously renewed attention focused on Mother Nature's pharmacy. New botanicals are being discovered all the time, like the rainforest herb cat's claw, or the pine bark ingredient pycnogenol, that have more powerful antioxidant properties than anything used during the past few decades to check free radical production. We are entering the "Phytochemical Revolution." The principal antioxidant players used in research so far have been vitamins C, E, and beta-carotene, and the minerals selenium, copper, zinc, and manganese (they are called the "mineral cofactors").

Research is now beginning to focus on the role of herbs as antioxidants, and new classes of herbs are emerging to categorize these specific actions.

During the past ten years, there has been increased research in the relationship between antioxidants and arthritis, allergies, chronic fatigue syndrome, cancer, AIDS, heart disease, infections, and numerous other illnesses. We have seen that phytonutrients are fast emerging as the preventive medicine of the future. Phytochemicals in foods and herbs are what has been the source of the folk remedies that our grandmothers knew about, but we, in our modern hustle and bustle, have forgotten. Today the therapeutic properties of these superfoods have been rediscovered and many have been found to be rich in antioxidant activity. In older herb books, "adaptogen," "immunomodulators," and "antioxidants" were not words given to describe the actions of herbs. But more modern herbals do include them, based on this growing body of research. Before we explore them, however, it may be helpful to examine just what the relationship is between antioxidants and free radicals.

There is scarcely a column on health and nutrition these days that doesn't mention these buzzwords. They are the subject of such immense interest because after at least thirty years, scientists and medical researchers have substantiated the theory that uncontrolled free radical production is the missing link between the origin and the progression of many diseases, hitherto thought to be unrelated. What's more, the nutritional research has uncovered a good body of evidence to validate the theory that free radicals can be effectively checked by phytonutrients, herbs, vitamins, enzymes, and other substances commonly called antioxidants.

What is a free radical? The simple answer is that it is an unpaired electron. Why is it so dangerous to a living organism? Free radicals develop within the human body and they also come from the environment. And they are not always the enemy! Our bodies make free radicals simply from the interaction between various substances and oxygen. Our immune systems make free radicals to destroy bacteria and viruses, to produce hormones, and to activate enzymes that regulate various chemical reactions that go on in the body. Clearly the free radical production that goes on inside each of us on a daily basis is not detrimental. However, when free radicals come from the environment, especially from pollution, tobacco smoke, toxic waste, pesticides, and radiation, a problem arises: When we inhale or ingest these substances, we get free radical overload.

When free radicals begin to multiply, a dangerous chain reaction begins to occur. The "radical" molecule must restore its balance by giving or taking an electron from another molecule. It is then said to be "reactive." When a molecule loses an electron, the process is called "oxidation." If allowed to multiply out of control, free radicals have one goal in mind: To pair at any cost. If not eliminated, the free radical activity will break off the cell membrane's proteins, thus destroying its identity; fuse together the proteins of the membrane, making it very brittle; or even puncture the membrane, making it vulnerable to disease-invading organisms. Once out of control, this reaction can open and destroy the nucleus of the cell, mutate and destroy its genetic material, and put undue stress on the immune system. Immune cells contain a high percentage of polyunsaturated fatty acids, which are especially prone to free radical invasion, therefore profoundly limiting the immune cell's ability to function in a healthy way.

There is a continual tug-of-war between the oxidation molecules and the antioxidants the body naturally produces. The process of oxidation is what causes food to turn rancid, metal to rust, or rubber to turn brittle. In the same way, unchecked oxidation has the potential to cause a great deal of damage to our cells, tissues, and organs. Our natural defense system produces antioxidants to come to the rescue. They do this by combining with and neutralizing the oxygen radicals, thus breaking the free radical chain. The body's first line of defense against radical oxidants are its enzymes, which require various minerals as cofactors. One of the most important antioxidant enzymes, for example, is superoxide dismutase (SOD), which is dependent on zinc and copper.

There are numerous nutrients that can boost immunity besides the antioxidants most of us are familiar with. These cofactors are vitally important. Folic acid, vitamin B6, copper, and magnesium are all involved in the formation of new cells, and a steady supply of these vitamins and minerals are essential in fighting off microorganisms that undermine a healthy immune system. Many herbs are rich in some of these minerals; and although it is best to get one's minerals from organic sources, some of these antioxidant minerals can be bought very cheaply at your local drug store.

Zinc, for example, is important in fighting off a variety of viruses, parasites, and other infectious diseases. The older we get, the more we need vital nutrients like this (which does not translate into taking huge doses of anything!). Many diets of the elderly fall short in specific nutrients necessary for optimum immune system functioning. Taking a multivitamin may not be a simple solution, because some nutrients need to be taken alone or in certain combinations in order to be effective. Iron, for example, prevents zinc absorption. So does calcium. Zinc is best taken on an empty stomach, generally, or with an SOD enzyme. SOD supplementation is one of the most effective free radical fighters available in oral form. Blue-green algae or wheat grass are excellent natural forms of this enzyme.

When we are exposed to excess environmental and psychological stress, we produce too many free radicals and disable our own antioxidant defenses: in short, we develop disease because we begin to lose the battle against free radicals, or perhaps we could say that we disrupt the balance because of free radical overload. The cells and tissues suffer what is called oxidative stress and the equilibrium is lost. As the power shifts to a series of free radical chain reactions, there is a kind of structural meltdown that begins to occur in the body part most subjected to the stress.

The effects of unchecked free radical damage by air pollution alone is extremely alarming. Nitrogen dioxide has been the culprit of many suspected lung disorders in people living in crowded cities. In Los Angeles, nearly 6,000 deaths per year are attributed to complications from breathing industrial soot spewed into the atmosphere. That is four times as many people that die every year from car accidents there. Continued exposure to air pollution increases the risk of inflammation in the lungs, especially among children. Asthma victims are at extremely high risk. One study showed that in a high smog area (Los Angeles), 80 percent of young people who had died in accidents had lung damage when autopsied.[1] Inhaled pollutants are not detoxified by the liver the way ingested pollutants are. They enter the bloodstream directly after being inhaled into the lungs. This is one reason why cigarette smoking is so damaging.

Radiation is particularly dangerous to the DNA and poses its own set of hazards. Radiation is a powerful carcinogen that severely depresses immunity. Some doctors believe that people who undergo radiation therapy are more likely to have their cancer metastasize to other parts of their body. Dr. John Cairns, quoted earlier, has stated that the majority of cancers are not cured by radiation because the dose needed to kill the cancer would also kill the patient.[2]

Ionizing radiation (frequently found in x-rays and gamma rays, nuclear reactor plants, and irradiated foods) and non-ionizing radiation (from too much sunlight, microwaves, power lines, and electrical appliances) all cause free radical damage. Radiation always induces a free radical process because it gives the chemical bond sufficient energy to tear it apart, thus releasing a single electron.

We also get free radical damage from unhealthy diets, especially diets high in polyunsaturated fats, which are more prone to oxidation than monounsaturated fats. Diets high in animal fat are more dangerous, not only because of cholesterol (still a controversial theory, at best) but because the chemicals that form free radicals from the environment are stored in an animal's fat cells. One major researcher in the antioxidant field, Steven Levine, has written that we now have "a proliferation of chemicals totally unprecedented in human evolution . . . [causing] oxidative stress to our bodies."[3]

A leading-edge researcher in this area, Dr. Debasis Bagchi of the Creighton University School of Pharmacy & Allied Health Professions, has said, "Free radicals have been implicated in over a hundred diseases in humans, including arthritis, hemorrhagic shock, atherosclerosis, aging, ischemia . . . gastritis, tumor promotion . . . and AIDS."[4]

Therefore, if oxidative stress becomes more than our bodies can handle, we must have additional defenses. Otherwise we risk becoming one of the statistics for many degenerative diseases that can lead to premature aging and death. In an overview of the current research, Nancy Bruning, an editor of *Natural Health Magazine,* summed it up: "[The] data is incriminating enough to convince many responsible researchers that free radicals could play a significant role in many disease processes that have puzzled us for centuries."[5] Some feel, in fact, that this research is opening up a field called the "Unified Disease Theory." As Bruning goes on to inquire, "Is it really possible that so many seemingly unrelated diseases—cancer, heart disease, chemical sensitivities, neurological disease, and arthritis—share the same common denominator: free radical damage?"[6] In addition, the question I would pose is: Is it really possible that we have so much free radical damage because we are exposed to 10,000 more chemicals than a short generation or two ago?

Some scientists estimate that the number of oxidative "hits" every day to human DNA per cell is more than 9,000. It is now believed that oxidative stress is a major player in heart disease. When the lining of blood vessels is damaged, the damage occurs not only to the lining but also to cholesterol molecules. Hundreds, if not thousands, of studies now associate low levels of vitamins A, C, and E with increased cardiovascular disease.

Dr. Hari Sharma, author of *Freedom from Disease: How to Control Free Radicals, A Major Cause of Aging and Disease,* has said that when we are exposed to excessive free radical proliferation, "the weakest link in the body will give way."[7] This is where antioxidants enter the picture. Antioxidants, in study after study, have been reported to capture free radicals before they attach to vital tissues. They help maximize cell defense. Frequently they work together; for example, vitamins C and E work as a team to control cell membrane damage. Oxidative stress always weakens the immune system. Antioxidants help to rebuild it. There is increasing evidence that the accumulation of free radical damage is what causes aging, and there may be a link between longevity and antioxidants. Certainly antioxidant supplementation has been shown to boost immune system functioning in the elderly in numerous trials. David Lin, in *Free Radical and Disease Prevention: What You Must Know,* explains:

[S]tudies suggest that the maximum number of years humans can live is 120. Few have approached that age and the majority become weak and ill much sooner. Perhaps by learning to control excessive free radicals, more of us will not only be able to live to 120 years, but do so in health and strength. In effect, we may be able to almost double our present life expectancy of 70 or so years and make them healthier and more productive.[8]

Of course, the Hunza, who live into the hundreds quite normally, are a living testimony to what we may all achieve if we could reverse the free radical overload with a healthy diet and environment. Interestingly, a 1997 article in *Newsweek* called "How To Live To Be 100" highlighted the notion that life expectancy continues to increase along with our changed attitude concerning it. Says Dr. John Rowe, a New York geriatrician who heads the Research Network on Successful Aging, "Until recently, there was so much preoccupation with disease that little work was done on the characteristics that permit people to do well."[9] Some of these measures include a more vegetarian-based diet, curbing free radical intake as much as possible, and a daily intake of antioxidants. The article, which reviewed a number of people who had lived to be a healthy 100, concluded that one of the reasons was that "by eating plants, you bathe yourself in cancer-fighting phytochemicals, bone-saving calcium, and the fiber needed to maintain a healthy colon and modulate blood sugar."[10]

One researcher, Richard Passwater, has demonstrated that several antioxidants administered to animals increased their average life span by 20 to 30 percent. His work, called *The Antioxidants: The Nutrients that Guard Us Against Cancer, Heart Disease, Arthritis, and Allergies, and Even Slow the Aging Process,* first published in 1985, was a summary of extensive research over many years. His more recent *The New Super-Antioxidant Plus* focuses on pycnogenol, a free radical antagonist that is more than fifty times more powerful than vitamin E and twenty times more powerful than vitamin C.[11] Pycnogenol and cat's claw are two of the major players emerging from the herb kingdom in fighting degenerative diseases. Other more traditional herbs that have long been used to strengthen the immune system are echinacea, hawthorn, ginkgo, ginseng, garlic, and milk thistle. These phytonutrients are so valuable I am including a separate section on their antioxidant and adaptogenic abilities; they are listed in my list of the twelve most important herbs in chapter 7. Numerous other phytonutrients that possess antioxidant properties can be found in the herbal part of this book and in the next chapter. See also the charts on antioxidant foods and herbs.

Foods are vitally important in terms of daily immunostimulant protection. Indeed, many foods and phytonutrients from foods are emerging in current research as vital protectors from cancer. Foods found to be most effective in avoiding cancer are: soy products, high fiber foods (especially yellow, orange, and green vegetables and fruits), and grains, which are rich in selenium. The foods that are richest in antioxidants are fruits and vegetables. It is probable, according to Dr. Bagchi, that the extremely high incidence of cancers in Central and Eastern Europe is due to high levels of pollution, fat, dairy, and meat consumption, coupled with low consumption of fiber, primarily from fruits and vegetables.[12]

Along with many others, Dr. Bagchi concludes that:

the potential role of antioxidant vitamins such as vitamin C, beta-carotene, and atocopherol, [vitamin E] antioxidant minerals such as zinc and selenium and antioxidant enzymes . . . have been extensively reviewed in the prevention of tumor growth and cancer.[13]

Some might object that taking food supplements every day may not be cost effective. But a closer examination of some of the key antioxidant players paints a picture that looks more like this:

Vitamin C from rose hips: 100 tablets, $7–8

Selenium: 60–90 tablets, $4–6

Zinc: 60–90 tablets, $5–6

Vitamin E: 90–100 softgels, $5–7

Mixed-carotenes or one bottle of
    carotene-rich blue-green algae: $8–10

Total average cost: $10–15 per month

Most of these supplements can be purchased at any local drugstore at comparable prices. Prices may increase slightly if obtained from sources that are organic. (See the next chapter for more organic sources of herbal minerals and antioxidants.) Regardless, compare this to the costs of surgery, doctor bills, hospital expenses, and other miscellaneous medical bills—not to mention time lost from work. Preventive health care, in my opinion, is always more economical.

Notes

1. D. B. Menzel, "Antioxidant vitamins and prevention of lung disease," *Annals of the New York Academy of Science* (30 September 1992), pp. 141–155.

2. J. Cairns, "The treatment of disease and the war against cancer," *Scientific American* (November 1985), p. 22.

3. S. A. Levine and P. M. Kidd, "Antioxidant adaptation: a unified disease theory," *Journal of Orthomolecular Psychiatry* 14, no. 1 (1984): 33.

4. D. Bagchi and S. K. Dash, "Environmental health, free radicals and antioxidants," *Townsend Letter for Doctors & Patients* (April 1997), p. 74.

5. N. Bruning, *The Natural Health Guide to Antioxidants* (New York: Bantam Books, 1994), p. 34.

6. Ibid., p. 52.

7. H. Sharma, *Freedom From Disease: How to Control Free Radicals, a Major Cause of Aging and Disease* (Veda Publishing, 1993), p. 74.

8. D. J. Lin, *Free Radicals and Disease Prevention: What You Must Know* (New Canaan, Conn.: Keats Publishing, Inc., 1993), p. 37.

9. In G. Cowley, "How to live to be 100," *Newsweek* (30 June 1997), p. 59.

10. Ibid., p. 64.

11. R. Passwater, *The Antioxidants: The Amazing Nutrients that Fight Dangerous Free Radicals, Guard Against Cancer, and Other Diseases, and Even Slow the Aging Process* (New Canaan, Conn.: Keats Publishing Group, 1985, 1997); *The New Superantioxidant-Plus: The Amazing Story of Pycnogenol, Free Radical Antagonist and Vitamin C Potentiator* (New Canaan, Conn.: Keats Publishing Group, 1993). See also his *Cancer Prevention and Nutritional Therapies* (New Canaan, Conn.: Keats Publishing Group, 1993.

12. Bagchi.

13. Ibid., p. 76.

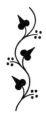

The idea is to live life more fully and more joyously.
—Dr. Dean Ornish

7

Latest Research on Adaptogens and Antioxidants

In this chapter, we want to examine only the adaptogen, antioxidant, and immunostimulant categories of certain nutrient-dense plants. Of course, herbs generally fall into numerous categories and the following herbs have a broad spectrum of action, which can be found in the herbal section of this book under the plant's name. For now, let us examine what is meant by these new ways of classifying phytonutrient herbs.

An adaptogen is any herbal agent that can help boost resistance to stress. Since new research indicates stress is one major cause of free radical formation, these herbs are particularly useful in exerting a balancing effect on the body, particularly the heart, nervous system, and immune system. Ways in which they enhance health include supporting the adrenals, improving blood sugar metabolism, flushing the liver, and stimulating antioxidant activity. In short, an adaptogen "normalizes" most any adverse condition in the body. In particular, they help us rebound from stress, thus improving stamina and endurance. However, a stressor is generally interpreted to mean anything that pulls the body out of balance, whether it be mental, emotional, physical, or chemical. Sometimes genetic factors predispose us to certain stressors. Whatever the cause, in my experience, the stress one is subjected to is much better tolerated when an adaptogen is taken on a daily basis. Many herbalists consider ginseng to be the best adaptogenic herb, and indeed it has long been revered as a tonic that heals everything. Personally, I think the most powerful adaptogenic food is algae or spirulina.

Antioxidants are sometimes classified as adaptogens, but they are more targeted to support the immune system and fight free radicals. Phytonutrients that are particularly rich in antioxidant properties are the bioflavonoids. The bioflavonoids can be found in many fruits and vegetables as well as herbs, and are especially useful in protecting against prostate and breast cancers, since they modify hormone receptors. Some of the richest bioflavonoid herbs are pine bark, grape seed, bilberry, ginkgo, hawthorn, and milk thistle. Antioxidant herbs are important in increasing the uptake of tissue oxygen, especially ginkgo and algae-based foods.

Immunostimulant is another word used to describe an herbal agent that enhances the body's defense systems. For example, echinacea and cat's claw are powerful immunostimulants that work by increasing the body's defense response through production of interferon or white blood cells. Some herbs, such as garlic, protect the immune system by their antibiotic or antibacterial action; that is, they kill or arrest the growth of pathogenic microorganisms.

Immunomodulators are agents that exert a positive effect on the immune system, or on a particular immune function. However, in some cases, they also have a negative effect—that is, a therapeutic suppression—of immune function. An example of this would be the suppression of immune function for treating organ transplant rejection or autoimmune disease. This is why they are called immunomodulators. Some of the most widely used herbs that fall into this category are the various ginseng roots and certain medicinal mushrooms, especially reishi.

Following is a list of what I consider to be the most important herbs that fall into these categories.

The Twelve Most Important Herbs

Algae, Spirulina, and Seaweeds

There are countless varieties of algae on our planet, often classified by their color: brown, green, red, blue-green. Wherever there is water, there is algae. They have sometimes been called the "lungs" of the earth, since algae is responsible for nearly 90 percent of all the oxygen we breathe. For centuries, coastal people all over the world have been eating sea plants; seaweeds are particularly popular among the Japanese, who have the highest longevity rate of any other culture (America ranks eleventh). Sea vegetables are excellent nutrients to purify, cleanse, nourish, and rebuild the entire body system. They alkalize the body and transform many toxins into harmless salts the body can dispose of. According to marine biologist Goran Michanek, the alginate in algae binds to heavy metals, which are then secreted from the body:

> The carbohydrates making up the algae cell walls are called alginate. Alginate has the unique and important ability of binding to heavy metals and radioactive substances to its own molecules. As the alginate cannot be broken down by bile or saliva, and cannot be absorbed by the body, it is secreted from the body together with the heavy metals and/or radioactive substances.[1]

Marine flora have been shown to possess numerous antioxidant, antimicrobial, and antibiotic properties, and many contain antitumor agents as well. They protect from cancers of the digestive tract by swelling in the intestines and diluting potential carcinogens; by cleansing the body of toxic waste; and by producing compounds that have been demonstrated in numerous studies to inhibit the growth of tumors. In particular, research supports the conclusion that seaweeds containing the active component, fucoidan, are associated with reduced breast cancer risk.[2] Other studies have shown that another constituent, the sulfolipids, protect human T cells from infection with the AIDS virus.[3] The immune-enhancing properties of chlorella have been observed to protect against cancers of the breast, blood, skin, and liver in animal tests.[4] Blue-green algae appears to be a strong protective agent against a number of microorganisms that cause disease. A team of researchers in Canada found that within two hours of eating 1.5 grams of algae, an average of 40 percent of the natural killer cells left the bloodstream and migrated to tissues, where their main function was to eliminate virally infected cells. These results, recently published, indicate that blue-green algae may be a valuable protection against both cancer and viruses.[5] No other substance is yet known to trigger such a powerful movement of NK cells (protective T cells) in the body.

Numerous sources indicate that Irish moss, kelp, and other seaweeds protect from radiation effects and reduce absorption of strontium, which is a radioactive isotope produced in some nuclear reactions and that is present in the environment. Green and blue-green algaes have been shown to have positive effects on brain functioning and learning disabilities.[6] The antioxidant beta-carotene, used in so many studies on free radical reduction, is very plentiful in blue-green algae. One study demonstrated that beta-carotene may be one of the major constituents in algae that is influential in removing cancer-causing free radicals.[7]

If you see a consistent theme that runs through these studies, so do I: It's called "protection." Algae products may be especially important for women. Rosemary Gladstar advises two tablespoons of spirulina a day for treating fibrocystic breasts, and also advises blue-green algae to maintain healthy breast tissue.[8]

I consider algae and spirulina to be the perfect food, with an abundant array of vitamins, minerals, and amino acids in a balanced and very assimilatible form. Most dried seaweeds can be kept in storage for years without losing their potency, which is another reason algae is at the top of my millennium medicine chest list.

Bilberry

Bilberry is another antioxidant herb that helps inhibit free radical damage in human tissue. Its active ingredient, anthocyanosides, is a vaso-protective agent. The early studies on bilberry began with anecdotal evidence of British pilots taking the herb (in jam) for better night vision. Bilberry has since been shown to have a positive effect on vascular integrity and in stabilizing blood capillaries. It leads to a reduction in capillary fragility and hemorrhaging.[9]

In Europe, the herb has become the most frequently prescribed medication for the treatment of eye disorders, as well as for the maintenance of healthy vision. It allows for adaptation to both light and dark, and is also good for eyestrain. Extracts of bilberry demonstrated antiviral properties for herpes simplex virus type 2, influenza, and certain kinds of bacteria, as well as viruses.[10] It has anti-inflammatory activity and may be effective in the prevention of thrombosis and angina. Very promising are the studies on its use an as anti-ulcer agent. Bilberry displays both preventive and curative properties in experiments with subjects who have ulcers.[11]

Women given bilberry extract during pregnancy had fewer varicose veins and circulatory problems.[12] Double-blind studies showed protective results in vascular disorders, especially in the lower limbs.[13] It is an excellent herb for circulatory problems in general associated with aging. Studies show it is also good for protection of connective tissue, as is the case with many of the bioflavonoids.[14] This makes it a useful adjunct for an herbal program treating arthritis, and research has demonstrated it also has anti-inflammatory properties for this condition.[15] This emerging research indicates that bilberry is a wonderful herb to add to one's diet to counteract many degenerative diseases associated with aging.

Cat's Claw

There is hardly a more remarkable herb to emerge (very recently) on the urban scene than cat's claw, or uña de gato, and it is stirring up much exciting research and expectation for the future. Its biologically active constituents have unique protective properties and it has been used as a wonder plant in its native land of Peru for centuries. The polyphenols in cat's claw make it a very powerful antioxidant and immunostimulant, and it has so many other healing characteristics—including those that help the body deal with stress—that it can also be classified as an adaptogen. Adaptogenic herbs are simply astonishing in their vast array of actions.

Present researchers are investigating cat's claw as a possible cure for certain kinds of cancer and AIDS. In a research laboratory in Austria, doctors have been experimenting with uña de gato since 1990 and it has shown remarkable results in retarding the progression of the AIDS virus. Currently an extract of cat's claw is being used in combination with the drug AZT in hopes of not only inhibiting the growth of HIV, but also in reducing the unpleasant side effects of AZT and radiation.[16] The bark contains alkaloids, which increase the ability of white blood cells and macrophages to attack, engulf, and destroy abnormal cells and inhibit the multiplication of viral agents.[17] Doctors in Peru have already been using it as a successful adjunct in the treatment of cancer.[18]

Cat's claw is also an anti-inflammatory, and it acts as a natural steroid. Its alkaloid content makes it a valuable aid in the treatment of arthritic conditions. I use it with black cohosh and just a little bit of ma-huang whenever I have an occasional arthritis flare-up and it works wonders. One isolated constituent, beta-sitosterol, appears to bind to cholesterol and prevent cholesterol absorption. Studies on heart health also show cat's claw having the ability to inhibit platelet aggregation and thrombosis—which are what causes blood to clot or get sticky (aggregation)—and may be valuable in the prevention of strokes.[19]

Dr. Donna Schwontkowski believes that cat's claw is the most powerful immune-enhancer ever discovered in the Amazon. She reports that uña de gato has decreased skin tumors and cysts within two weeks; that it has been linked with the remission of brain and other tumors; that it is a helpful adjunct in offering relief from the side effects of chemotherapy; that it has helped fight infections in AIDS patients; that it offered relief for patients who are chemically sensitive; and that it has been helpful in relieving the symptoms of gastritis, ulcers, arthritis, and wounds.[20]

Another researcher of this amazing herb, Dr. Brent Davis, who has been evaluating cat's claw since 1988, has said that in his opinion its therapeutic implications far surpass other world-class herbs, such as echinacea, goldenseal, ginseng, and astragalus, because it has more immunologically active constituents than any other single herb.[21] So far, at least six have been identified. However, most researchers believe that the activity of the whole plant extract is greater than the sum of its parts. Dr. Davis has also said that cat's claw has an amazing ability to detoxify the intestinal tract and treat a variety of stomach and bowel disorders. He refers to the herb as "the opener of the way" because of its remarkable efficacy in breaking through severe intestinal derangement, such as leaky gut syndrome, which no other products are able to do as effectively.[22]

Cat's claw is a woody vine that grows to over 100 feet in length. Most of the highly active components in cat's claw are found in the inner bark, and since the bark can be harvested without the destruction of the whole plant, it can be used without the danger of destroying the Amazon ecosystem.

So far, the properties attributed to cat's claw include adaptogenic, antioxidant, anti-inflammatory, antimicrobial, antiviral, and antitumor. Keep your eyes open for new developments on this amazing jungle herb.

Cayenne

Cayenne is not actually a pepper; peppercorn is a seasoning entirely different from this species of vegetable, and has little redeeming nutritional value. Cayenne, or capsicum, has long been an important remedial herb, imported into the West from India in the late fourteenth century. Its name, from the Greek, means "to bite," an allusion to its hot, pungent nature. Its healing properties are so numerous that Dr.

Christopher included it in his list of the ten most important herbs. It has been popular among herbalists traditionally because it was thought to improve circulation, fight fatigue, stimulate blood flow to the brain, equalize and strengthen heart and nerves, aid in digestion, and rejuvenate and cleanse the entire body. Cayenne stimulates circulation, thereby increasing the oxygen exchange capacity of the lungs and acting as a catalyst in blood purification. It insures the rapid and even distribution of the active principles in other herbs with which it is combined.

According to Frances Albrecht, president of Nutrition Education Services at Bastyr University, the capsaicin in cayenne keeps toxic chemicals from attaching to DNA, where they can trigger changes that lead to lung and other cancers.[23] Cayenne inhibits the excess production of a chemical called Substance P in the body, which is involved with the transmission of pain impulses. Because the activity of cayenne targets this particular kind of chemical reaction, one of its principal chemical uses has been in the form of a skin emollient for the treatment of fibromyalgia, diabetic neuropathy, and other forms of chronic pain. Double-blind studies have been performed indicating that such nerve pain associated with diabetes is significantly reduced.[24] It is also instrumental in reducing arthritis, lumbago, and other rheumatic pains, especially when applied topically.[25]

Tests with human subjects with rhinitis show promising results in reducing nasal obstruction and secretions.[26] Cayenne aids in the digestion and assimilation of food and has been used successfully for flatulent dyspepsia (imperfect or painful digestion).[27] Also, when used properly, cayenne can help eliminate ulcers. In *The Scientific Validation of Herbal Medicine,* Dr. Daniel Mowrey suggests that the controversy over whether cayenne cures or causes ulcers is directly related to its use. Under certain conditions—that is, when applied directly to inflamed tissues and combined with a high-fat, low-protein diet, it may damage mucosal cells and cause an ulcer. However, administration in low doses with adequate nutrition has produced hundreds of cayenne-induced ulcer cures.[28]

Finally, research has now begun to focus on cayenne's use as an agent to lower blood serum cholesterol, especially when combined with hawthorn.[29]

Curcumin (Turmeric)

Could an ancient spice be important in the future for treating cancer, arthritis, and heart disease? A component of curry powder has produced tantalizing possibilities in numerous laboratory tests that indicate the answer may be yes. Curcumin, the phytochemical that lends the yellow-orange color to the root powder in turmeric, is the substance attracting much current attention. Turmeric has long been used in India and Southeast Asia as a natural remedy for inflammation and digestive disorders. Only recently has it come to the attention of modern researchers, who continue to unfold newer, and quite astonishing, developments in the study of this aromatic spice from the East.

Its antimutagenic properties are presently being investigated. A number of studies have demonstrated that curcumin can shut down the mechanisms responsible for cell proliferation. "An enormous amount of literature supports the anticarcinogenic and anti-inflammatory properties of curcumin," according to Bharat Aggarwal of the University of Texas Anderson Cancer Center in Houston.[30] Dr. Aggarwal's group has found that curcumin has the potential to block tumor metastasis, or the spread of cancer normally responsible for death. In numerous experiments the treatment with this ancient herb reduced the number of tumors in mice that were exposed to a known carcinogen, and the tumors that did develop were less likely to be invasive.[31] It appears to act both as an antioxidant and as an inhibitor of a lipid called prostaglandin, responsible for inflammation and tumor promotion.

Turmeric exhibits cardiotonic activity as well, including the ability to inhibit platelet aggregation (stickiness), which may be one reason why thrombosis is much less likely to occur in countries where this spice is used regularly. It also prevents the rise of serum cholesterol.[32]

A 1991 review of the pharmacology of curcumin also confirmed its long use as an antibacterial and antifungal agent.[33]

Although the bulk of cancer research has been done with animals, the treatment of arthritis sufferers with turmeric has focused on human subjects. In one double-blind study, the patients given the herb instead of a placebo showed a significant lessening in the severity of pain and mobility of movement.[34] Like other anti-inflammatory agents that do not contain steroids, curcumin appears to work by strengthening the adrenals.[35]

Turmeric has traditionally been used as a cholagogue, or liver tonic. Like milk thistle, curcumin increases the secretion of bile and, when combined with milk thistle, potentiates its cholagogue effect by more than 300 percent.[36] More recent studies suggest that curcumin can help in the prevention of cataract formation.[37] It appears that turmeric is too much of an anticoagulant in some people, and it should not be taken with anticlotting drugs.

Echinacea

Echinacea is one of the favorite remedies in my herbal medicine chest. In this era of renewed interest in natural methods of living and healing, it is also an herb that is enjoying great popularity. It is most noted for its action as an antiviral, antifungal, and natural antibiotic. It is one of the herbs considered to be a blood purifier. This category of herbs does not imply that they scrub your blood in some magical way, but that they stimulate blood flow through the liver, thus aiding in clearing out toxins.

Echinacea has long been available in Europe as an over-the-counter supplement for prevention and treatment of colds and flu, as well as for vaginal yeast infections, bronchitis, and ear and sinus infections. It was an extremely common herbal remedy in the early American development, when eclectic, or "alternative," medicine was as popular as "traditional" medicine is today. When the schisms within the medical disciplines began to erupt in the early part of this century, the AMA published negative reports on echinacea and, in its mania to "clean up" the profession, eventually triumphed in its stranglehold on American health care. Echinacea fell out of popularity and all writing and research in the medical literature on it ceased abruptly in the mid-1930s. It was not until the 1970s that echinacea was reintroduced to the U.S. by manufacturers from Europe.

The polysaccharides in echinacea activate the body's immune system, increasing the activity of white blood cells and producing interferon, which is important in protection from viral infections. However, the extract of echinacea, unlike the drug interferon, remains active when stored at room temperature. Thus, extracts of echinacea can be stored indefinitely and used when necessary. Many studies have been done on human subjects with both colds and flus that point to the herb's effectiveness to curtail symptoms and duration of infections as well as preventing their recurrence.[38]

As an immune stimulant, echinacea appears to work best when taken in measured periods of time, apparently to prevent building up resistance to the herb. Some herbalists feel it is contraindicated for use with autoimmune illnesses like lupus or multiple sclerosis, and possibly HIV. Research is still young in this area, however.

Because of its interferon-stimulating activity, echinacea is now being studied as a possible agent in the treatment of cancer and herpes.[39] Researchers have discovered a tumor-inhibiting principle in the oil that may protect against carcinosarcoma and leukemia.[40] Echinacea is also effective against candida (the yeast responsible for a painful vaginal infection for which antibiotics are often ineffective), as well as other vaginal infections.[41] Finally, clinical studies support the herb's use an anti-inflammatory for arthritis, which unlike steroids, does not suppress the immune system.[42] This makes steroids a poor choice for treating any inflammatory condition that needs a strong immune response.

Both *Echinacea angustifolia* and *Echinacea purpurea* (the type common to the U.S.) are equally effective. This humble plant—commonly known as purple coneflower—is thus emerging as one of the most powerful immunostimulants on the scene today, reaffirming its early use by both Native Americans and early American settlers as an excellent choice for fighting infection and building immune strength.

Garlic

Garlic has a long history as a plant food, known to the ancient Egyptians and mentioned in the Bible as well. It enjoys great popularity in the Mediterranean countries still, where the low incidence of heart disease has caused researchers to study its role in the circulatory system. There have been more than 900 scientific studies in the past twenty years documenting its many medicinal uses. (Only a few of them are included here!)

Garlic is a powerful activator of liver detoxification enzymes. One of its principle constituents, the thiols, block enzymes that promote tumor growth, particularly in the colon, lung, stomach, and esophagus. A study conducted by the National Cancer Institute demonstrated that people who included garlic and onions in their daily diets lowered their risk of stomach cancer by 40 percent. The allicin in garlic appears to protect against cancer by "waking up enzymes inside cells that detoxify cancer-causing chemicals."[43]

Garlic possesses both antimutagenic and antiviral properties. The extract has been shown to offer protection from staph and strep. The allicin in garlic and onions block the activity of toxins produced by countless other bacteria and viruses as well. It is estimated that one milligram of allicin is equal to approximately fifteen standard units of penicillin.[44] Allicin also increases the levels of two important antioxidant enzymes in the blood, catalase and glutathione peroxydase.

The two antioxidant minerals, selenium and organic germanium, are abundant in garlic and easily assimilated in the body. It may prove useful in the prevention of breast cancer.[45] Garlic is fast becoming America's number one choice as a natural alternative for lowering cholesterol and reducing blood pressure. Sales of garlic supplements are growing yearly by more than 100 per cent, and sales of garlic are also increasing.[46] Studies show garlic lowers cholesterol and triglycerides, inhibits platelet aggregation (stickiness), reduces blood coagulation and lowers blood pressure.[47] Most research indicates that 600–900 milligrams of garlic per day is necessary in lowering cholesterol.[48]

Garlic is truly a wonder food that I have used therapeutically for almost thirty years. I remember when living on a Missouri Ozarks farm, very isolated from access to doctors, I used garlic to treat a serious infection my son had as a baby. On the advice of a local herbalist, I taped garlic cloves to his feet and he recovered within twenty-four hours.

Garlic protects the liver from damage caused by chemical pollutants and synthetic drugs, and is an excellent antioxidant for all cellular membranes. A clove wrapped in gauze and inserted into the vagina is also good for minor female infections.

Unfortunately, the principle protective agent, allicin, is difficult to get from garlic supplements, since it is not very stable and is generally available only in macerated garlic oil products, not in garlic powder. The allicin is most available when eaten raw. Try it chopped in salads. Then plan to stay in for the evening!

Ginkgo Biloba

Although widely used in Europe for decades, one of the exciting new antioxidants emerging on the scene in the U.S. is the bioflavonoid ginkgo. At the time of this writing, close to 400 studies have used this herb and interest continues to grow in the general public as its sales increase almost weekly. Ginkgo is attracting a lot of attention from the baby boomers who want very much to stave senility, not only by keeping fit but also by nurturing the brain. Ginkgo biloba appears to be one of those brain foods, demonstrating relief from memory impairment and increased ability to concentrate.[49] It may even emerge as an aid for Alzheimer's disease in the future. Perhaps there is a mystique surrounding the herb because the ginkgo tree lives to be a healthy 1,000 years old, and is the world's oldest living species of tree. No wonder claims are being made about it staving Alzheimer's disease and preserving memory! Whether it holds up to these claims in the future remains to be seen.

What is quite clear is that ginkgo increases the quantity of capillary circulation, thus increasing blood flow to the brain, heart, and other organs.[50] The bioflavonoids, combined with the terpene components, not only improve circulation but also help prevent platelet stickiness and protect from atherosclerosis.[51] This increased blood flow to the brain may be what is successfully reversing depression in some elderly patients.[52] Studies show the antioxidant properties of ginkgo appear to protect the retina, and it may be useful for eye disorders such as cataracts and macular degeneration, a leading cause of adult blindness.[53]

One interesting study found that it prevented radical damage to the kidney and liver caused by immunosuppressive drugs used in transplants.[54] It may prove valuable in the future to prevent the rejection of transplanted organs. Much of ginkgo's healing potential is connected to its suppression of what is called the platelet activation factor (PAF), which is related to organ graft rejection, asthma attacks, and blood flow through the arteries. One study found that ginkgo was the most potent PAF inhibitor of the components tested in relieving bronchoconstriction due to asthma and allergic inflammation.[55] It may prove to be a valuable aid in stroke prevention since it appears to protect nerve cells in the central nervous system from damage during periods of ischemia.[56] A TIA, or transient ischemic attack, is a severe lack of blood flow to body tissues, and is generally a warning sign for stroke. Ginkgo seems to be particularly effective for pain in the legs due to poor circulation.[57] Its PAF-inhibiting action may not be well suited, however, for people with clotting disorders.

All considered, ginkgo biloba is a remarkable herb and has been safely used by much of the world's population for hundreds of years. Even if it does not turn out to be a panacea for preserving memory or curing Alzheimer's disease, I believe it is a valuable herb to take daily for its powerful antioxidant properties.

Ginseng

The three principal types of ginseng are Panax (or Asian), American, and Siberian. Ginseng is a remarkable adaptogen and immunomodulator. My favorite ginseng is eleuthero, or the Siberian variety, although technically it is not considered to belong to the ginseng family. It does, however, have similar effects, and is often used interchangeably with the Panax or Asian variety. Ginseng has been used traditionally to invigorate the body as well as calm the spirit. It has long been believed that ginseng improves mental and physical performance and aids in any kind of debility. In the East, it is prized for promoting longevity and increasing resistance to disease.

In terms of studies, there are many. Ginseng is perhaps the most well-researched herb on earth, yet how it works is still something of a mystery. Many make claims that ginseng is a panacea (hence the name "Panax") for nearly everything; others believe it is worthless. (The traditional hype about ginseng as an aphrodisiac has not been supported by research.) Most medical research seems to suggest that its unusual power as an adaptogen tends to have contradictory effects. For example, in some people, ginseng may raise blood pressure; in others, it may lower it. Likewise, it may treat both diabetes (high blood sugar) and hypoglycemia (low blood sugar.) This is part of the nature of its balancing effect.[58]

Some adaptogens like ginseng fall into a preventive category, rather than targeting specific disease conditions. It is excellent for any kind of stress since it helps restore adrenal function. Siberian ginseng has been routinely used by Russian cosmonauts to improve endurance and responsiveness.[59] In contrast, American astronauts were offered artificial amphetamines. One research team investigated the effects of eleuthero used by Russian cosmonauts, Olympic athletes, and divers, and found that it consistently increased stamina and endurance.[60]

Ginseng is frequently found in herbal formulas designed to support the adrenals, because it allows them to function optimally under stressful conditions. The adrenals are extremely important glands of the endocrine system, which are responsible for producing some of the most vital hormones in the body. When the body labors under and kind of stress (physical or mental), the homeostasis—the balance and harmony within the body—is affected. Therefore, many people believe that taking ginseng as a daily supplement is helpful, especially if one is experiencing stress on a regular basis. (And in this day and age, who isn't?)

Ginseng has been shown to ameliorate the effects of radiation exposure. Rats exposed to radiation damage lived twice as long when given ginseng, with less damage to blood and tissue. It increases resistance to radiation by as much as 500 percent.[61] Some of the victims of the Chernobyl nuclear disaster were given Siberian ginseng to help with this antiradiation effect. It also is an aid in reducing the side effects of radiation and chemotherapy.[62] Oncology clinics in Russia and Germany have used it extensively. Ginseng has been demonstrated to improve immune function in numerous studies.[63] It increases the number of T lymphocytes as well as the natural killer cells. There is also a rise in the concentration of blood corticoids, leading to an improved resistance to infections.[64] As an immunomodulator, it may be a useful adjunct in therapy for AIDS, cancer, chronic fatigue syndrome, and autoimmune disorders.

In my mind, adaptogens are gifts from the Creator to help modify the effects of environmental stresses like chemical pollutants, radiation, and poor diet, as well as emotional and other internal stresses so prevalent in our world today.

Milk Thistle

Milk thistle is often called the liver herb, and it is vital to first understand how valuable this organ is before one can appreciate the actions of this antioxidant. The liver is involved with so many other physiological processes that it is impossible to enumerate them all. However, a few very important ones are the metabolism of carbohydrates and the maintenance of blood sugar; the correct metabolism of proteins; the synthesis of cholesterol; the storage and use of vitamins; and the detoxification of drugs, pollutants, food additives, poisons, and radiation. It is essential for maintaining healthy blood, gallbladder, digestion, and endocrine function.

If the liver is not functioning optimally, it may manifest as any variety of symptoms in the body; for example, skin disorders. There has probably never been a time in human history when the liver has been as taxed as it is today. I imagine it like a tired but ceaselessly dedicated worker doing a lot of overtime to rid the body of pollutants.

Dr. Michael Murray, in his *21st Century Herbal,* has suggested that the standardized extract silymarin, combined with curcumin, offers powerful antioxidant protection to keep the liver functioning optimally in our stressful and polluted world.[65] They protect the liver from chemical damage and improve liver function in experimental and clinical studies.[66] Milk thistle apparently works by protecting the outer membranes of liver cells, by scavenging free radicals, and by regeneration of damaged or injured liver cells.[67] It increases the very important SOD enzyme in red blood cells and produces another antioxidant, glutathione, in liver cells.[68] It is especially necessary for people with chemical sensitivities or those continually exposed to toxins in the work place. Studies indicate it will also ward off damage done by excessive use of alcohol or use of antidepressant or anticonvulsive drugs.[69]

Another study found that silymarin offers some protection against the toxicity of acetaminophen when taken over a long period of time.[70] The extract of milk thistle is the most important antidote to poisoning by the amanita ("deathcap") mushroom.[71] Dr. Murray advises it for treating hepatitis, psoriasis, and any condition in which the liver has been overburdened with poisons.[72] Milk thistle accelerates the regeneration of destroyed liver tissue by stimulating protein synthesis. In studies where the livers of rats were partially removed, the administration of silymarin regenerated it.[73] The American Liver Foundation has issued a report that hepatitis C is greatly on the increase and is expected to triple within the next decade, reaching almost "epidemic proportions."[74] Four and one-half million people now have it, and it is a disease that takes years to develop. This is a vital herb to keep around in the future!

It may even be useful as a protection from the effects of chemotherapy.[75] Taken in high doses, however, it may cause loose stool, and it should not be used if there is a blockage of bile flow.

Pycnogenol

The Maritime pine is the magical tree credited with saving the lives of the famous explorer Jacques Carter and his crew when they were trapped on the St. Lawrence River in the winter of 1534. With no fresh fruits and vegetables, they were dying of scurvy by the droves until some friendly Indians fed the remaining crew tea from the bark of this plentiful pine. It cured them of scurvy and 400 years later we are discovering that this rich antioxidant, pycnogenol, is again restoring lives to wholeness.

Pycnogenol is not one specific nutrient, but rather a group of substances found in certain kinds of bioflavonoids. The most superior kind of bioflavonoid, in terms of its antioxidant properties, are called proanthocyanidins, found abundantly in pine bark and grape seed. Because the body cannot produce bioflavonoids, they must be supplied daily through diet or supplements. The proanthocyanidins are particularly helpful in stabilizing collagen structures, which hold tissue together.[76] The regular use of pycnogenol thus aids in maintaining flexibility of joints and surrounding tissues.

The grape seed bioflavonoids are antioxidants that prevent the oxidation of low-density lipoprotein, which offers protection against coronary heart disease.[77] Grape seed is a powerful inhibitor of free radicals and brings on a potentialization of vitamin C. In vitro tests show that, as a free radical scavenger, pycnogenol is fifty times more effective than vitamin E.[78] This is not to say that this will translate in exactly the same way in humans, but these studies are very promising. The bioflavonoids in pine bark and grape seeds have been found to be useful in treating dysfunctional capillaries, peripheral vascular diseases, varicose veins, and bruises, as well as numerous forms of tissue degeneration, including multiple sclerosis, muscular dystrophy, and Parkinson's disease.[79]

Like other adaptogens, pycnogenol has a large range of effects. Its antioxidant action slows cell mutagenesis (protecting from cancer) and its antistress actions helps prevent ulcer formation by 82 percent.[80] It improves the elasticity and general appearance of the skin. Pycnogenol is easily assimilated when taken orally, even in people with problems with assimilation, and it is also the only flavonoid that is known to cross the blood-brain barrier. Because of its rapid and easy assimilation, it is often effective when other free radical scavengers are not effective due to malabsorption.

Like Saint John's Wort, the powerful antioxidant effects of the proanthocyanidins come in deep colors. One researcher summed up the effects of this remarkable bioflavonoid:

> [They] are chemicals of intensely colored, sap-soluble glycoside plant pigments responsible for most scarlet, purple, and blue coloring in higher plants . . . [with] a radical scavenger effect which quenches pathology and stops deterioration in the 80 trillion cells in the body and brain.[81]

I eat my grape seed every day. Although most of the tests have been done using pycnogenol, I always prefer the safer, more holistic approach of using the whole herb. If taking pycnogenol, the dosage for general support is 50 milligrams; for therapeutic purposes, do not exceed 150 milligrams.

Saint John's Wort

Although the media coverage for Saint John's Wort has focused almost exclusively on its use as a Prozac substitute, there are many other useful applications for this herb. As an antioxidant, antiviral, anti-inflammatory, and antibacterial, Saint John's Wort has so many healing actions that it deserves our close attention in the future. Research is now beginning to focus, for example, on using Saint John's Wort to control the spread of the AIDS virus.

Researchers in both the U.S. and Israel have discovered that the standardized extract, hypericin, has potential antiviral activity.[82] Studies were first done on a retrovirus in mice, who do not get HIV. Since it inhibits a retrovirus in vivo (in animal studies), further research was done on the retrovirus HIV. Although these latter studies have principally used the extract in vitro (in test tubes), the preliminary results are astonishing. Hypericin has demonstrated an ability to prevent uninfected T lymphocytes from being infected by the HIV-1 virus.[83] Anecdotal reports from some individuals using the standardized dosage of hypericin also show promise, although the results are mixed and much more research needs to be done.[84] Some of the benefits of Saint John's Wort may be indirect, i.e., connected to its antidepressive effect, since it is known that depression directly suppresses immune function.

The antiviral components in these studies with Saint John's Wort are hypericin and pseudohypericin, while the proanthocyanidins are the constituents with the antioxidant and antimicrobial properties.[85] The antibacterial activity of the oil of Saint John's Wort has long been revered as a potent wound healer, and modern research supports this.[86] The oil is advocated by Rosemary Gladstar as the best remedy for herpes.[87] It reduces skin damage from radiation and offers relief from nerve and muscle pain. Its anti-inflammatory properties also make it an effective aid for muscle spasms, back pain, arthritis, and sciatica pain.

The oil of Saint John's Wort is bright red and looks like blood. Interestingly, according to the Doctrine of Signatures (an ancient belief that plants had been "signed" by God with some visible clue pointing to its therapeutic use), it was believed that this was the signature of Saint John's Wort, indicating its usefulness in treating wounds and blood disorders. It has traditionally been used as an alternative, or blood purifier. (Other actions of this marvelous herb can be found in the herbal part of this book.)

Saint John's Wort has become popular as an alternative to drugs such as Prozac and Zoloft, which are overprescribed and overpriced, and which have long-term accumulative side effects. For an excellent overview of the frightening research of long-term use of these dangerous antidepressants, see Ann Tracy's book *Prozac: Panacea or Pandora?*[88] This research is an excellent examination of the political evolution of the technology behind the production of these drugs, as well as the repercussions of the drugs themselves. Prozac, Zoloft, and Paxil should never be taken over an extended period of time, especially when there are alternatives like Saint John's Wort. In Germany, Saint John's Wort is the most popular antidepressant, outselling Prozac seven to one.[89]

Saint John's Wort is believed to alleviate depression and anxiety by inhibiting the neurotransmitter norepinephrine. Although the early studies attributed these effects to the hypericin, it is now thought to be a much more complex interaction.[90] Most Saint John's Wort extracts are standardized to contain measured amounts of hypericin; in the future, this may prove to be one of the downfalls of standardization. Saint John's Wort, even though acting as an MAO inhibitor, does not act like the class of Prozac drugs in other ways. Pharmacologists are still at a loss to explain how it does work. "We've tried to understand it by comparing it to the antidepressants we know, fitting it into the boxes we already have on the shelf, and so far it doesn't fit," said one pharmacist at the National Institute of Mental Health.[91]

Despite the fact that we still do not understand how it works, the herb continues to unfold new potential. Studies have shown it has potent antiviral properties for the Epstein-Barr virus, and some health-care practitioners are using it as an adjunct in the treatment of chronic fatigue syndrome.[92] One of my clients, who has chronic fatigue, has found that Saint John's Wort proved to be more effective than anything else. I feel that Saint John is a valuable ally and use it on occasion, especially in the wintertime. This herb, like any antidepressant, should not be taken indefinitely or thought of as a cure. If using it for depression, however, it is recommended that a dosage of 300 milligrams be taken three times a day (900 total). I have noticed that many formulas do not contain this amount of Saint John's Wort, but the synergistic effects of the other ingredients, as in the Dr. Christopher formulas, may augment the total effect. It is difficult to say, since these kinds of dosages have never been subjected to systematic testing. Hundreds of reports that I have received from my consulting over the past two years, however, indicate that they do indeed work. As an occasional mild sedative before bed, I find the tea to be an excellent relaxing brew.

Proper labeling should accompany Saint John's Wort and its formulas, especially if taken in high doses. It should not be taken with pickled foods, wine, weight-loss products, decongestants, other antidepressants or stimulants, like ma-huang. Light-skinned people may be at risk for blistering, and should not sunbathe when using the herb.

Finally: The Minerals!

Don't forget to boost your immune system with mineral-rich herbs! Here is an excellent formula that provides the full array of minerals (mineral cofactors) so necessary to supplement good antioxidant activity.

Combine equal parts of red clover, raspberry, dandelion, rose hips, parsley, yellow dock, and alfalfa. Pour boiling water over all, made with distilled water. Cover in a glass jar and shake often over a twenty-minute period. Strain. It may be drunk hot or cold. Enjoy!

Notes

1. G. Michanek, "Ocean Algae's Beneficial Effects," available from Westport Scandinavia, 3040 Valencian Ave., Aptos, CA.
2. K. Chida and I. Yamamoto, "Antitumor activity of a crude fucoidan fraction prepared from the roots of kelp (laminaria species)," *Kitasato Arch. of Exper Med.* 60, no. 1–2 (1987): 33–39; J. Teas, "The dietary intake of laminaria, a brown seaweed, and breast cancer prevention," *Nutrition & Cancer* 4 (1983): 217–22.
3. K. R. Gustafson, et al., "AIDS-antiviral sulfolipids from cyano-bacteria (blue-green algae)," *Journal of the American Cancer Ins.* 81, no. 16 (1989).
4. Y. Miyazawa, et al., "Immunomodulation by a unicellular green algae (chlorella pyrenoidosa) in tumor-bearing mice," *Journal of Ethnopharmacology* 24, no. 2–3 (1988): 135–146; I. Yamamoto, et al., "Antitumor activity of crude extracts from edible marine algae against L-1210 leukemia," *Botanica Marina* 15 (1982): 455–457.
5. G. S. Jensen, et al., "Effects of the blue-green aphanizomenon flos-aquae on human natural killer cells," *Phytoceuticals: Examining the health benefit and pharmaceutical properties of natural antioxidants and phytochemicals,*

IBC Library Series 1911, chapter 3.1, reproduced by Cell Tech; See also G. E. Zhukova, et al., "Inactivation of some RNA-contained viruses with green and blue-green algae," *Vestn. Mosk. Univ. Biol. Pochvoved* 27, no. 4 (1972): 108; O. Hayashi, "Enhancement of antibody production in mice by dietary spirulina platensis," *Journal of Nutritional Science and Vitaminology* 40, no. 5 (October 1994): 4431–41.

6. P. Tompkins and C. Bird, *Secrets of the Soil* (New York: Harper & Row, 1989), see chapter 18.

7. P. Nair, et al., "Evaluation of chemoprevention of oral cancer with spirulina fasiformes," *Nutrition and Cancer* (1995), pp. 197–202. See also *The Lancet* 346 (July 8, 1995): 75–81.

8. R. Gladstar, *Herbal Healing for Women* (New York: Simon & Schuster, 1993), pp. 155, 157.

9. A. Scharrer, et al., "Anthocyanosides in the treatment of retinopathies," *Klin Monatsbi Augenheilkd Beih* 178 (1981): 386–89; L. Caselli, "Clinical and electroretinographic activity of anthocyanosides," *Archi. Med. Int.* 3 (1985): 29–35.

10. M. Weiner, *Herbs That Heal* (Mill Valley, CA: Quantum Books, 1994), p. 84; A. E. Guinness, *Family Guide to Natural Medicine* (New York: Reader's Digest Association, 1993), p. 324.

11. A. Cristoni, et al., "Antiulcer and healing activity of Vaccinium myretillus nathocyanosides," *Farmaco, Edizione Practica* 42, no. 2 (1987): 29–43.

12. G. L. Grismond, "Treatment of pregnancy-induced phlebopathies," *Minerva Gynecol.* 33 (1981): 221–30.

13. G. Spinella, "Natural anthocyanosides in treatment of peripheral venous insufficiency," *Archi. Med. Int.* 9 (1985): 21–29.

14. J. C. Monbiosse, et al., "Non-enzymatic degradation of acid-soluble calf skin collagen by superoxide ion: Protective effect of flavonoids," *Biochem Pharmacol.* 32 (1983): 53–58.

15. C. N. Rao, et al., "'Influence of bioflavonoids on the collagen metabolism in rats with adjuvant induced arthritis," *Italian Jour. of Biochemistry* 30 (1981): 54–62.

16. R. Cerri, "New quinovic acid from uncaria tomentosa," *Journal of Natural Medicine* 51, no. 2 (March–April, 1988): 257–61; see also Philip Steinberg's *Cat's Claw News*, P.O.B. 1078, Washington, MO, 63090.

17. R. Aquino, et al. "Plant metabolites: structure and in vitro antiviral activity of quinovic acid glycosides from uncaria tomentosa," Journal of Natural Products 52, no. 3 (May–June, 1990): 559–564; P. Steinberg, "Uncaria tomentosa (Cat's Claw): A wondrous herb from the Peruvian rainforest," *Townsend Letter* 130 (May 1992): 2.

18. *New Editions Health World Magazine*, Feb. 1995, p. 43. See also Steinberg, above.

19. Aquino et al., "Plant metabolites, new compounds and anti-inflammatory activity of uncaria tomentosa," Journal of Natural Products 54, no. 2 (March–April 1991): 453–459; *Arthritis News* 1 (Summer 1989); J. Chen, et al., "Inhibitory effects of rhynchophylline on platelet aggregation and thrombosis," *Acta Pharmacologica Sinica* 13, no. 2 (1992): 126–30.

20. D. Schwontkowski, "Herbal treasures from the Amazon," *Healthy and Natural Journal* 1 (October 1994): 64-65.

21. B. W. Davis, "A new worldclass herb for A. K. practice: uncaria tomentosa," *Collected Papers of the International College of Applied Kinesiology*, Summer 1992.

22. B. W. Davis, *Cat's Claw News* (May/June 1995).

23. F. Albrecht, "The new generation of antioxidants," Nutrition Advisor, *Delicious Magazine* (March 1997), p. 74; See also A. K. Y. De & J. J. Ghosh, "Short and long-term effects of capsaicin on the pulmonary antioxidant enzyme system in rats," *Phytotherapy Research* 3, no. 5 (1989).

24. K. M. Basha, et al., "Capsaicin: A therapeutic option for painful diabetic neuropathy," *Henry Ford Hospital Medical Journal* 39, no. 2 (1991): 138–140.

25. G. Buzzanca & S. Laterza, "Clinical trial with an antirheumatic ointment," *Clin. Trials* 83, no. 1 (October 1977): 71–83. See also N. Jancso, et al., "Direct evidence for neurogenic inflammation and its prevention by denervation and by pretreatment with capsaicin," *British Jour. Pharmacol.* 31 (1967): 138.

26. S. Marabii, et al., "Beneficial effects of intranasal applications of capsaicin in patients with vasomotor rhinitis," *European Archives of Oto-Rhino-laryngology* 218, no. 4 (1991): 181–84.

27. H. Glatzel, "Blood circulation effectiveness of natural spices," Med. Klin. 62, no. 51 (December 1967): 1987–1989; H. Glatzel, "Treatment of dyspeptic disorders with spice extracts," *Hippokrates* 40, no. 23 (December 1969): 916–919; T. Koloata & D. Chungcharon, "The effect of capsaicin on smooth muscle and blood flow of the stomach and intestine," *Siriraj Hospital Gazette* 24 (1972): 1405–18.

28. D. Mowrey, *The Scientific Validation of Herbal Medicine* (New Canaan, Conn.: Keats Publishing, 1986), p. 295.

29. K. Sambaiah and N. Satyanarayana, "Hypocholesterolemic effect of red pepper and capsaicin," *Indian Jour. of Exper. Biology* 18 (1980): 898-99; see also P. Holmes, *The Energetics of Western Herbs* (Boulder, Colo.: Artemis Press, 1989).

30. *Women's Health Advocate Newsletter* 4, no. 8 (October 1997): 1.

31. Ibid. See also M. Nagabhushan and S. Bhide, "Antimutagenicity and anticarcinogenicity of turmeric (Curcuma longa)," *Journal of Nutrition, Growth and Cancer* 4 (1987): 83–89; K. Polassa, et al., "Turmeric (Cur-

cuma longa) induced reduction in urinary mutagens," *Food and Chemical Toxicology* 29, no. 10 (1991): 699–706.

32. H. P. Ammon & M. A. Wahl, "Pharmacology of Curcuma longa," *Planta Medica* 57, no. 1 (1991): 1–7; R. Srivastava, et al., "Effects of curcumin on platelet aggregation and vascular prostacyclin synthesis," *Arzneimittel-Forschung* 36, no. 4 (1986): 715–717 in D. Mowrey, *Herbal Tonic Therapies* (N.Y.: Wings Books, 1993).

33. See Ammon, *Pharmacology* . . .

34. D. Chandra and S. S. Gupta, "Anti-inflammatory and antiarthritic activity of volatile oil of Curcuma Longa (haldi)," *Indian Jour. of Medical Res.* 60, (1972); R. R. Kulkarni, et al., "Treatment of osteoarthritis with a herbomineral formulation: a double-blind, placebo-controlled, cross-over study," *Journal of Ethnopharmacology* 331, no. 1–2 (1991): 91–95.

35. R. Arora, et al., "Anti-inflammatory studies on curcuma longa (turmeric)," *Indian Journal of Experimental Biology* 56 (1971): 1289–95; N. Ghatak and N. Basu, "Sodium curcuminate as an effective anti-inflammatory agent," *Indian Jour. of Exp. Biology* 10 (1972): 235–236.

36. S. Zaterka and M. I. Grossman, "The effect of gastrin and histamine on secretion of bile," *Gastroenterology* 50 (1966): 500.

37. See #1, above.

38. H. Wagner and A. Proksch, "Immunomodulatory drugs of fungi and higher plants," in N. Farnsworth, H. Hikino, and H. Wagner, eds., *Economic and Medicinal Plant Research Vol. 1*, (Orlando, Fl.: Academic Press, 1985), pp. 113–155; H. Wagner, "Immunologically active polysaccharides from tissue cultures of Echinacea purpurea," proceedings from the Thirty-fourth Annual Congress on Medicinal Plant Research, Hamburg, Sept. 22–27, 1986; D. Shoneberger, "The influence of immune-stimulating effects of pressed juice from Echinacea purpurea on the course and severity of colds," *Forum Immunologia* 8 (1992): 2–12.

39. J. L. Hartwell, "Plants used against cancer: A survey," *Lloydia* 32 (1969): 247–296; D. J. Voaden and M. Jacobson, "Tumor inhibitors 3: Identification and synthesis of an oncolytic hydrocarbon from American coneflower roots," *Jour. of Medicinal Chemistry* 15 (1972): 619; A. Wacker and W. Hilbig, "Virus-inhibition by Echinacea purpurea," *Planta Medica* 33 (1978): 89–101; C. Lersch, et al., "Stimulation of the immune response in outpatients with hepatocellular carcinomas by low doses of cyclophosphamide, echinacea purpurea extracts and thymostimulin," *Archiv fur Geschwulstforschung* 60, no. 5 (1990): 379–83, cited in D. Mowrey, *Echinacea* (New Canaan, Conn.: Keats Pub., 1995).

40. D. J. Voaden and M. Jacobson, "Tumor-inhibitors III. Identification and synthesis of an oncolytic hydrocarbon from American coneflower roots," *Journal of Medicinal Chemistry* 15, no. 6 (1972): 619–623.

41. E. Coeuginiet and R. Kuehnast, "Recurrent candidiasis: adjuvant immunotherapy with different formulations of echinacin," Therapiewoche 36, no. 33 (1986): 3352–58; in D. Mowrey, Echinacea (New Canaan, Conn.: Keats Pub., 1995). See also C. Hobbs, "Echinacea: A literature review," HerbalGram 30 (1994): 33–48.

42. E. Tragini, et al., "Evidence from two classic irritation tests for an anti-inflammatory action of a natural extract, echinacea B," Food and Chemical Toxicology 23, no. 2 (1985): 317–319.

43. F. Albrecht, "The new generation of antioxidants," Nutrition Advisor, Delicious Magazine (March 1997), p. 74; see also S. Belman, "Onion and garlic oils and tumor protection," Carcinogenesis 4 (1983): 1063–65; E. Dorant, et al., "Garlic and its significance for the prevention of cancer in humans: A critical view," British Jour. of Cancer 67 (1993): 424–429; R. McCaleb, "Anticancer effects of garlic—more proof," HerbalGram 27 (1992): 22–23.

44. C. J. Cavallito and J. H. Bailey, "Allicin, the antibacterial principle of allium sativum," Journal of the Amer. Chemical Society 66 (1945): 1950–51; L. Jezowa, et al., "Investigations on the antibiotic activity of allium sativum," Herba Polonica 12, no. 3 (1966); K. Nagai, "Experimental studies on the preventive effect of garlic extract against infection with influenza virus," Japanese Jour. of the Assoc. for Infectious Diseases 47 (1973): 111–115.

45. S. Weed, Breast cancer? Breast Health! (Woodstock, N.Y.: Ash Tree Pub, 1996); see also C. Ip, et al., "Mammary cancer prevention by regular garlic and selenium enriched garlic," Nutrition & Cancer 17 (1992): 279–286.

46. K. Deveny, "Garlic pills are potent drugstore sellers," Wall Street Journal 1 October 1992.

47. R. Gebhardt, "Multiple inhibitory effects of garlic extracts on cholesterol biosynthesis in hepatocytes," Lipids 28 (1993): 613–619; J. Kleijnen, et al., "Garlic, onion and cardiovascular risk factors. A review of the evidence from human experiments with emphasis on commercially available preparations," British Jour. of Clin. Pharmacol. 28 (1989): 535–544; A. Bordia and H. C. Bansal, "Essential oil of garlic in prevention of atherosclerosis," The Lancet 11 (1973): 1491; C. Silagy and A. Neil, "Garlic as a lipid lowering agent—a meta-analysis," The Jour. of the Royal College of Physicians 28, no. 1; M. Chi, "Effects of garlic products in lipid metabolism in cholesterol fed rats," Proceedings of the Society for Experimental Biology and Medicine 171 (1982): 174–78.

48. "Herbal Immunity Boosters," a report from the Herb Research Foundation (No author given), Fall 1995, p. 15. Published by the Herb Research Foundation, 1007 Pearl St., Boulder, Colo.

49. G. Voberg, "Ginkgo biloba extract (GBA): A long termstudy of chronic cerebral insufficiency in geriatric patients," Clinical Trials Journal 22 (1985): 149–157; G. S. Rai, et al., "A double-blind placebo controlled study of

Ginkgo biloba extract in elderly outpatients with mild to moderate memory impairment," *Current Med. Research Opin.* 12 (1991): 350–355.

50. F. Clostre, "From the body to the cellular membranes: The different levels of pharmacological action of Ginkgo biloba extract," in E. W. Funfgeld, ed., *Recent Results in Pharmacology* (Berlin: Springer-Verlag, 1988), pp. 180–198; see also P. Braquet, ed., *Ginkgolides: Chemistry, Biology, Pharmacology and Clinical Perspectives* Vol. 2 (Barcelona: J. R. Prous Science Publishers, 1989).

51. K. F. Chung, et al., "Effect of a ginkgolide mixture in antagonizing skin and platelet responses to platelet activating factor in man," *The Lancet* (31 January 1987).

52. I. M. Lesser, et al., "Reduction in cerebral blood flow in older depressed patients," *Arch. Gen. Psychiatr.* 51 (1994): 677–686.

53. C. Ferrandini, M. T. Droy-Lefaix, and Y. Christen, eds., *Ginkgo biloba Extract as a Free Radical Scavenger* (Paris: Elsevier, 1993).

54. S. A. Barth, et al., "Influences of Ginkgo biloba on cyclosporin A induced lipid peroxidation in human liver microsomes in comparison to Vitamin E, glutathione and N-acetylcysteine," cited in M. Weiner and J. Weiner, *Herbs That Heal* (Mill Valley, CA: Quantum Books, 1994), p. 166.

55. P. Braquet and D. Hosford, "Ethnopharmacology and the development of natural PAF antagonists in therapeutic agents," *Jour. of Ethnopharmacology* 32, no. 1–3 (1991): 135-39.

56. J. Krieglstein, "Neuroprotective properties of Ginkgo biloba constituents," *Phytotherapy* 15 (1994): 92-96.

57. B. Schneider, "Ginkgo biloba extract in periphreal arterial disease: Meta-analysis of controlled clinical trials," *Arzneim-Forsch Drug Research* 42 (1992): 428-36.

58. "Herbal Immunity Boosters," a report from the Herb Research Foundation (No author given), Fall 1995, published by the Herb Research Foundation, 1007 Pearl St., Boulder, Colo.; N. R. Farnswoth, et al., "Siberian ginseng: current status as an adaptogen," in H. Wagner, et. al, eds., *Economic and Medicinal Plant Research, Vol. 1* (London: Academic Press, 1985), 155–215.

59. S. Fulder, "The drug that builds Russians," *New Scientist* (21 August 1980).

60. Brekhman, II, *Man and Biologically Active Substances* (Oxford: Pergamon Press, 1980).

61. "Herbal Immunity Boosters," a report from the Herb Research Foundation (No author given), Fall 1995, published by the Herb Research Foundation, 1007 Pearl St., Boulder, Colo., p. 10; see also D. Tenney, *Ginseng* (Pleasant Grove, Utah: Woodland Publishing, 1996).

62. E. Ben-Hur and S. J. Fulder, "Effect of ginseng saponins and eleutherococcus on survival of cultured mammalian cells after ionizing radiation," *American Jour. of Chinese Medicine* 9 (1981): 48–56; See also R. J. Collisson, "Siberian ginseng (Eleutherococcus sentiosus)," *British Jour. of Phytotherapy* 2 (1991): 61–71; K. V. Yarameko, "The main aspects of the use of Eleutherococcus extract in oncology," in *New Data on Eleutherococcus and other Adaptogens* (Vladivostok, USSR: USSA Academy of Sciences, 1981), pp. 75–78.

63. B. Bohn, et al., "Flow-cytometric studies with Eleutherococcus senticosus extracts as an Immunomodulatory agent," *Arzneimittel-Forschung* 37, no. 10 (1987): 1193–96.

64. S. J. Fulder, "Ginseng and the hypothalamus-pituitary control of stress," *American Jour. of Chinese Medicine* 9 (1981): 112–118; V. K. Singh, et al., "Immunomodulatory activity of Panax Ginseng extract," *Planta Medica* 50 (1984): 462–465.

65. M. Murray, *The 21st Century Herbal* (Bellevue, WA: Vita-Line, Inc., 1996).

66. H. Wagner, "Plant constituents with antihepatotoxic activity," in J. L. Beal and E. Reinhard, eds., *Natural Products as Medicinal Agents* (Stuttgart: Hippokrates-Verlag, 1981); J. E. Reynolds, ed., *Martindale: The Extra Pharmacopoeia* (London: Pharmaceutical Press, 1982).

67. D. Brown, *Introduction to PhytoTherapy* (New Canaan, Conn.: Keats Pub., 1995).

68. G. Muzes, et al., "Effect of the bioflavonoid silymarin on the in vitro activity and expression of superoxide dismutase (SOD) enzyme," *Acta Physiol. Hungarica* 78 (1991): 3–9; A. Valenzuela, et al., "Selectivity of silymarin on the increase of the glutathione content in different tissues of the rat," *Planta Medica* 55, no. 5 (1989): 420–22.

69. R. Ferenci, et al., "Randomized controlled trial of silymarin treatment in patients with cirrhosis of the liver," *Jour. of Hepatology* 9 (1989): 105–13; E. Leng-Peschlow, "Alcohol related liver diseases—use of Legalon for therapy," *Pharmedicum* 2 (1994): 22–27; see also G. Palasciano, et al., "The effect of silymarin on plasma levels of malondialdehyde in patients receiving long-term treatment with psychotropic drugs," *Current Ther. Res.* 55 (1994): 537–45.

70. R. Campos, et al., "Silybin dihemisuccinate protects against glutathione depletion and lipid peroxidation induced by acetaminophen on rat liver," *Planta Medica* 55 (1989): 417–19.

71. M. Murray, *The 21st Century Herbal* (Bellevue, WA: Vita-Line, Inc., 1996), p. 30.

72. Ibid., pp. 26–30.

73. D. Mowrey, *Herbal Tonic Therapies* (N.Y.:Wings Books, 1993), p. 226.

74. CNN report, 5 March 1998.

75. S. Weed, *Breast Cancer? Breast Health!* (Woodstock, N.Y.: Ash Tree Pub., 1996), p. 278.

76. R. Passwater, *The New Superantioxidant Plus: The Amazing Story of Pycnogenol* (New Canaan, Conn.: Keats Pub., 1992), p. 14.

77. B. Schwitters and J. Masquelier, *OPC in Practice: Bioflavonoids and Their Application* (Rome, Italy: Alfa Omega, 1993); M. G. Hertog, et al., "Dietary antioxidant flavonoids and risk of coronary heart disease: the Zutphen Elderly Study," *The Lancet* 342 (1993): 1007–11.

78. See Passwater, #76. See also M. Walker, "Medical journalist report of innovative biologics: Antioxidant properties of pycnogenol," in *Townsend Letter for Doctors* (August/September 1991), pp. 616–17.

79. Ibid., Walker. See also J. Masquelier, "Pycnogenols: recent advances in the therapeutic activity of procyanidins," *Journal of Medicinal Plant Research* (July 1980), pp. 243–56.

80. D. Bell, International Symposium on Pycnogenol, Bordeaux, France (October 1990) and S. Brown, International Symposium on Pycnogenol, Bordeaux, France (October 1990) in R. Passwater, *The New Superantioxidant Plus: The Amazing Story of Pycnogenol* (New Canaan, Conn.: Keats Pub., 1992); see also "Inflammation and nutrition," *Anon. Medical Nutrition* (Autumn 1989), pp. 42–45.

81. M. Walker, "Medical journalist report of innovative biologics: Antioxidant properties of pycnogenol," in *Townsend Letter for Doctors* (August/September 1991), pp. 618.

82. D. Meruelo, et al., "Therapeutic agents with dramatic antiretroviral activity and little toxicity at effective doses: Aromatic polycyclic diones hypericin and pseudohypericin," *Proceedings of the National Academy of Sciences* 85 (1988): 5230–34.

83. G. Lavie, et al., "Studies of the mechanism of action of the antiretroviral agents hypericin and pseudohypericin," *Proceedings of the National Academy of Sciences* 86 (1989): 5963–67; J. B. Hudson, et al., "The importance of light in the anti-HIV effect of hypericin," *Antiviral Research* 20 (1993): 173–178.

84. J. James, "Hypericum: Common herb shows antiretroviral activity," *AIDS Treatment News* 63 (1988): 1–5. See also J. James, "Hypericin results: Community Research Alliance study," *AIDS Treatment News* 96 (1990): 2–4.

85. "Herbal Immunity Boosters," a report from the Herb Research Foundation (No author given), Fall 1995, published by the Herb Research Foundation, 1007 Pearl St., Boulder, Colo.

86. M. K. Saka and A. U. Tamer, "Antimicrobial activity of different extracts from some Hypericum species," *Fitoterapia* 61 (1990): 464–66.

87. R. Gladstar, *Herbal Healing for Women* (New York: Simon & Schuster, 1993), p. 148.

88. A. Tracy, *Prozac: Panacea or Pandora?* (Cassia Pub., 1994)

89. B. Carey, "The sunshine supplement," *Health* (January/February 1998), pp. 52–56.

90. V. H. Muldner and M. Zoller, "Antidepressive effect of hypericum extract standardized to the active hypericin complex: Biochemistry and clinical studies," *Arzneim-Forsch Drug Research* 34 (1984): 918–20; J. Holzl, et al., "Investigations about antidepressive and mood changing effects of Hypericum perforatum," *Planta Medica* 55 (1989): 643; G. Harrer and H. Sommer, "Treatment of mild/moderate depressions with Hypericum," *Phytomedicine* 1 (1994): 3–8.

91. B. Carey, "The sunshine supplement," *Health* (January/February 1998), p. 54.

92. H. Someya, "Effect of a constituent of Hypericum erectum on infection and multiplication of Epstein-Barr virus," *Jour. Tokyo Med. Coll.* 43 (1985): 815–26; L. Rector Page, *Herbal Pharmacist,* 1991. Published by the author. See p. 67.

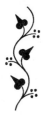

*Technology and the incredibly rich tapestry it has
made possible has created a false sense of security . . .
the thread is flawed. The tapestry is now fragile.*

—GERI GUIDETTI

8

A Millennium Herbal
First-Aid Kit

As we sit on the edge of the next millennium, we face many unknown challenges; indeed, many of us believe that the earth itself seems to be going through some kind of major change. What this bodes for the future remains to be seen, and I am not going to spend much time here conjecturing. However, we so often take for granted the conveniences of modern life that many of us would not know how to survive in a natural environment should the need arise that would force us to do so. Dr. Christopher believed that an emergency herbal first-aid kit should be in every home or car. I personally feel that every home should also have a stock of at least twenty-five to fifty herbs, as well as dried foods and pure water, in the event of a natural (or not-so-natural) disaster. But maybe that's just because I live in California, and earthquake preparedness is often on Californians' minds. Nonetheless, as we begin the new millennium, I feel that many prophecies, as well as numerous news stories, are quietly warning us that we should be prepared for any possibility that may develop in the future that would force us into total self-reliance; in other words, in which a doctor or hospital may not be available.

This may seem farfetched to some, but it is always a possibility. An herbal medicine chest is especially important for people who have chosen not to live in cities. I raised my son in the southern Missouri Ozarks, where the closest doctor or hospital was eighty miles away. So I am well aware that herbal first aid is a vital necessity for many. We often take for granted the conveniences of modern life, and many of us would not have a clue as to how to survive in a natural environment, should the need arise that would force us to do so.

The original subtitle for this book was "A Millennium Medicine Chest;" and the reason I spent as much time doing the research I did for the chapters preceding the herbal part of this book is that I believe it is of utmost importance that we become self-reliant enough to survive in the face of impending crises, be it personal or global. In any event, for those interested in herbal emergencies, I have included this section. It has some useful remedies, most of them given to us by Dr. Christopher. The following first-aid formulas should hopefully get you busy collecting things to make your own herbal first-aid kit!

An Herbal First-Aid Kit

Wounds, Abrasions, and Infections
Arnica; calendula; comfrey; plantain (see part II, the herbal, for specifics on each herb)

Arnica ointment is excellent for immediate external application. Calendula oil is soothing for scratches, bruises, sprains, and dry skin. Comfrey will help stop bleeding and prevent infection; take it internally and make a poultice or compress for application on the skin. Fresh or powdered comfrey can also be applied directly to wounds. Plantain is an astringent and antiseptic and may be used both internally and externally.

Burns

Aloe; tea tree oil; Saint John's Wort oil; Dr. Christopher's comfrey ointment

Keep a live aloe plant nearby and apply as needed. Slice leaves and use directly on the skin. Tea tree oil is difficult to make and impossible to grow in the U.S. However, I suggest you keep a commercial jar in storage at all times. It is one of the most powerful antiseptics and healers for burns and infections from burns. Use Saint John's Wort oil for application on wounds, burns, and skin exposed to radiation (see the herbal for specifics on Saint John's Wort). Here is how to make Dr. Christopher's comfrey paste: Mix honey and wheat germ oil in equal parts. Blend in finely chopped or powdered comfrey (root, leaf, or a combination) until the mixture is a heavy paste. Apply directly to burn area, cover with gauze, and bandage lightly. When paste has been absorbed, add more on top of it; do not remove original.

Broken Bones

Oatstraw; Saint John's Wort; skullcap; comfrey

Drink infusions of oatstraw copiously. It is rich in calcium. Mix it with comfrey tea as well for a powerful nutritive herbal drink for bones. Use Saint John's Wort oil on the area that is mending if the bones are in a splint. (Bones heal better in a splint rather than in a cast.) Drinking Saint John's Wort tea and absorbing the oil through the skin will help healing and also prevent nerve damage. Take skullcap teas and tinctures to ease pain and calm anxiety or induce sleep. Make a comfrey fomentation: Pour boiling water over leaves; soak a towel in the infusion; cover area and wrap with plastic.

Colds, Flu, and Congestion

Yarrow; echinacea; peppermint; boneset

Yarrow is excellent mixed with peppermint for the sniffles. Use echinacea to rebuild immune strength. Drink the tea, tincture, or keep powdered echinacea on hand to cap as needed. Take boneset tea to bring down fevers and help alleviate mucus. Boneset leaves should steep, covered, in a hot place for thirty minutes. It may be mixed with yarrow.

Indigestion, Nausea, and Stomach Problems
Catnip; licorice; peppermint; ginger

Catnip tea is useful for colic or indigestion; it has a natural antacid effect. Licorice will help heal the mucous membranes of the stomach and cure chronic conditions of indigestion. Peppermint tea is helpful in many kinds of stomach upset and will ease nausea or morning sickness almost immediately. Ginger is good to eat often after a meal to aid in digestion. Dried ginger, which can be stored for years, is easily reconstituted.

Earaches
Garlic; mullein; chamomile; lobelia

Use 4–6 drops of garlic oil directly in the ear; plug with a cotton ball. Likewise, mullein oil may be used the same way, or a combination of the two oils used together in equal parts. To make garlic or mullein oil, crush herb, soak in olive oil, and put in a warm place (such as a radiator or warm oven) for several hours until the oil of the herb is extracted into the olive oil. Strain; discard the solid material. Or, make a fomentation of 3 parts chamomile and 1 part lobelia; soak a towel in the infusion and squeeze directly in the ears. Also, drink chamomile tea every 2 hours until pain subsides. Chamomile is very safe to drink copiously. It may be mixed with skullcap (see broken bones) to help ease pain and calm anxiety.

Fungal Infections, Ringworm, and Skin Diseases
Black walnut; tea tree oil; goldenseal; myrrh

Use black or English walnut in a tincture form, both externally and internally, three times daily. Or, apply tea tree oil directly to the fungal area; use frequent applications. An infusion can be made of equal parts goldenseal and myrrh, and also applied directly to the skin as long as condition persists.

Bites and Insect Repellent

Black or English walnut; pennyroyal; plantain; marshmallow

The oil of black or English walnut and pennyroyal are both effective as bug repellents. Pennyroyal oil may be diluted with lard and brushed around the baseboards of the home. A plantain leaf or powder placed over a bite or sting will often bring relief. Marshmallow acts as a natural antihistamine. (See part II, the herbal, for more specifics.)

Toothache

Clove oil

Apply directly onto tooth cavity.

Sprains and Muscle Cramps

Cayenne; comfrey; white willow; Saint John's Wort

Make a cayenne healing liniment in emergencies by massaging cayenne tea, tincture, or oil into the affected body part. Wash hands thoroughly after use. Cayenne is very potent and should be used in a proportion of 1:8 to other oils or ointment preparations. For best results, stock up on Dr. Christopher's capsicum healing balm. Or make a comfrey paste (see above, under burns or check the herbal for poultice). Use white willow and Saint John's Wort for pain and inflammation.

Recovery From Any Disease or Infection

Garlic; cayenne; ginseng; echinacea

Garlic and cayenne will help fight infections and kill pathogens. Ginseng will rebuild strength and help the body adapt to stress. Echinacea will build the immune system back up, fight free radicals, and facilitate overall healing. In acute conditions, echinacea should be taken every 2 hours. Do not exceed 10 days.

A General Germicide

This can be used for sterilization of any skin tissue surface: Mix equal parts of goldenseal, myrrh, comfrey root, garlic, and cayenne in 40 percent pure grain alcohol. Close lid tightly. Keep jar in a warm place for several weeks if possible, shaking well twice a day. Strain and seal. Use when necessary.

For Immediate Food Source When Real Food Is Not Available

Algae; licorice; ginseng; alfalfa

See the section of blue-green algae and seaweeds in chapter 7. Algae is one of nature's most perfect foods, containing every known nutrient. The powder form keeps indefinitely. Licorice is an excellent herb to rebuff hunger and thirst. The armies of Alexander the Great carried the root with them on their long journeys for strength and stamina. It feeds the adrenals directly and sustains energy. Ginseng is also a valuable energy herb that helps to balance blood sugar. Alfalfa is a powerhouse of vitamins and minerals. If fresh food were not available, one could exist indefinitely on powdered capsules of the above nutrients and pure water.

PART II

Alfalfa

Buffalo herb, purple medic

Alfalfa is a common field perennial with erect smooth stems that grow as high as two feet. It is a member of the legume family, with spiral seed pods and trifoliate leaves. The flowers are blue, purple, or yellow, and are clustered around the central stem.

Parts used: Leaves, sprouts

Therapeutic Profile

Alternative
Diuretic
Galactagogue
Tonic
Anti-inflammatory
Nutritive

Recent Research

The high nutritive value of alfalfa has been verified by numerous laboratory tests. It has also been shown to lower cholesterol and to retard the development of diabetes in mice.

Medicinal Uses; Catalysts and Combinations

Alfalfa is an excellent tonic, especially for the stomach. It not only has a very high nutritional value, but it is useful in treating both acute and chronic digestive weaknesses. It has many trace minerals and enzymes so essential for good health and also aids in the assimilation of proteins. The herb has long been used as an aid for arthritic and rheumatic pains. It is a good diuretic for acute cystitis and will increase milk secretion in nursing mothers. It is an extremely potent source of chlorophyll, a good infection fighter, and a natural mouth deodorizer. It stimulates removal of inorganic mineral deposits and will counteract the development of ulcers. Complementary agents include juniper, marshmallow, and buchu.

Dosage and Administration

Use approximately 1 ounce of dried leaves to 1 pint of water. Steep 10 minutes and drink hot or cold as often as desired. Tablets and sprouts may be eaten as a dietary food supplement.

Gathering and Useful Notes

Harvest alfalfa as the flowers bloom. Cut plants back and leave the stem to continue growing; then hang to dry. Always keep some seeds on hand for easy sprouting. Exert caution if you eat copious amounts of the sprouts, as it may induce blood abnormalities in some people. The tea is very safe and nutritious.

History and Lore

In folklore, alfalfa was believed to help solve money problems. It was also worn in an amulet for protection. Alfalfa is an ancient remedial herb, mentioned as far back as 3000 B.C.E. by the Emperor of China. However, early Western herbalists like Grieve do not seem to have noticed it. Most likely, it was not an herb that attracted much attention, since it was believed to be a simple tonic, primarily nutritive rather than medicinal. The ancient Arabs called alfalfa the "father of all foods." Spanish explorers brought it to the New World and it eventually took root and became the most popular plant for cattle feed.

Correspondences

    Planet: Jupiter
    Element: Fire
    Gender: Male
    Sign: Sagittarius

Aloe

Barbados aloe, aloe vera, cape aloe, burn plant

Aloe has a strong, fibrous root that produces fleshy leaves up to two feet long. It is light green on both sides with spiny teeth on the edges. The plant is cool to the touch, and is gelatinous when the leaves are split open. It has yellow or purple flowers.

Part used: Interior of leaf

Therapeutic Profile

Cholagogue
Laxative
Demulcent
Vulnerary

Recent Research

The fresh leaf enhances healing of wounded cells and promotes growth of normal cells in laboratory and clinical settings. Studies show the juice increases absorption of food, protects against bacteria and yeast, and heals ulcers. It is immune-enhancing and may prove useful for viruses such as HIV and herpes.

Medicinal Uses; Catalysts and Combinations

Aloe promotes cell regeneration of wounds. Taken as a juice, it acts as a mild laxative, and also heals gastritis. It is a healing agent for infections and fungal skin conditions. Mixed with juice, it is a digestive tonic. There are testimonies for its positive effect on arthritis. In creams, it counteracts wrinkles and may help regulate female hormones. It has also been used in the treatment of frostbite. It has antioxidant effects to help combat radiation and airborne pollutants.

It combines well with fennel to counteract the effect of griping (cramping), and with turmeric for regulation of liver function. Aloe may stimulate menses and should not be taken during pregnancy.

Dosage and Administration

Split the leaf and apply directly to cuts and burns. Drink 4–12 ounces a day for stomach problems, or a dose of 1–5 grams may be taken daily in capsule form, especially for gastritis or ulcers. In tincture form, take 5–30 drops.

Gathering and Useful Notes

Do not harvest immature plants or use younger plants for household burns. Plants should have 3–5 years of growth. Always harvest outer leaves first. Discard soon, as the leaves become rancid. It must be dried carefully; some studies show dry aloe is not nearly as effective as the fresh.

History and Lore

History tells us aloe was used by Alexander the Great for healing the wounds of his soldiers. Scientific validation of its wound-healing properties dates from the 1930s, when it was noticed that the gel hastened the healing of x-ray burns. It has been used medicinally in India for at least 3,500 years, and was a common medicine among the American Indians, who called it the "Wand of Heaven." It has long been regarded as a funeral herb, being planted on graves to bestow peace until the Resurrection; Nicodemus, who was at the tomb of Christ, brought with him a mixture of myrrh and aloe. It has the reputation of bringing success into one's life and was often hung over doorways for protection, or worn by travelers. Aloe is called *kumari* in Sanskrit, which means "goddess."

Correspondences

Planet: Moon
Element: Water
Gender: Female
Sign: Cancer

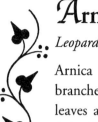

Arnica

Leopardsbane, wolfsbane, mountain arnica

Arnica has a brown rootstock with a hairy or lightly branched stem, growing to a height of one to two feet. The leaves are oblong, and the flowers are large, yellow, and daisy-like.

Parts used: Flowers, root

Therapeutic Profile

Anti-inflammatory
Analgesic
Vulnerary

Recent Research

Chemical studies have isolated a number of constituents that are anti-inflammatory and antibiotic.

Medicinal Uses; Catalysts and Combinations

Arnica is primarily used as an ointment for injuries and bruises. It is an excellent soothing salve for rheumatic and inflammatory pain. It reduces swelling, and is helpful in the treatment of phlebitis and shingles. It may be used as a poultice for abdominal pain. As a lotion, it combines well with witch hazel. A dilute tincture can be made for inflammations of the mouth, but it generally should not be taken internally except in homeopathic preparations.

Dosage and Administration

The commercially available tincture is easy to find; it may be used freely as oil or liniment. To make your own, see below. Do not take internally.

Gathering and Useful Notes

Flowers are collected when they bloom, from June through August, and dried. To make a tincture, pour 1 pint of alcohol over 2 ounces of flowers, and seal for a week in the sun. To make an oil, macerate flowers in olive oil, leave three days, and strain through a cloth. It may be used in massage or herbal baths.

History and Lore

Arnica has been used by both European and American Indian cultures for centuries. Many drug preparations in Europe still incorporate it for its analgesic effects. American Indians taught the use of arnica salve for stiffened muscles and wounds to the white settlers. It is not to be confused with elecampane, called "false arnica."

Correspondences

Planet: Saturn
Element: Earth
Gender: Female
Sign: Capricorn

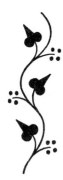

Astragalus
Huang chi; tragacanth

Astragalus is an herb common to China. It has stems and stout branches with ten to twelve small leaves on each branch, and yellow flowers budding at the top.

Parts used: Root or whole plant

Therapeutic Profile
Adaptogen
Diuretic
Mucilage
Immunostimulant
Tonic

Recent Research
Exciting research shows that astragalus stimulates the proliferation of white blood cells. Cancer patients display greater immune response than controls, and it may prove useful in the treatment of AIDS.

Medicinal Uses; Catalysts and Combinations
Extracts of astragalus have demonstrated antibacterial effects, and it is gaining wide interest as a powerful immune strengthener. It is an organ toning and balancing herb, and can be used as a diuretic for kidney inflammations. It appears to be effective against the papillomavirus virus and herpes simplex virus type 2. It is good for peripheral vascular diseases and influenza. It combines well with a Chinese herb called ligustrum as an immune enhancer. As a thick mucilage, it can be used with most liniment formulas.

Dosage and Administration

Use 1 teaspoon of root to 1½ pints of water. Drink 1 cup twice daily for immune protection, unless under the supervision of a health-care practitioner for treatment of more severe problems.

Gathering and Useful Notes

If using the root for tea, boil slowly for 30 minutes, then allow to cool slowly in a closed container. It may also be mixed with other kinds of herbs for a poultice effect; use 2 ounces of mucilage with 3–4 teaspoons of the dried herb.

History and Lore

Astragalus is a popular herb in China, which has a very long history of herbal cures. It is revered for its natural defense against disease. It has been called "wind energy" because it overcomes fatigue and is an overall body tonic. The recent research in using astragalus in cancer treatment has led to a new understanding of the relationship between traditional Chinese medicine and Western medicine. Used as an adjunct to chemotherapy, the 4,000-year-old Chinese herbal tradition of using astragalus is proving highly effective in strengthening the immune system and reducing tumors. Chinese medicine has been in existence for thousands of years and modern physicians are beginning to realize that there must be some value to this time-honored tradition. In the West, astragalus has been tested for its immunomodulating activity and has been found to increase white blood cells.

Correspondences

Planet: Mercury
Element: Air
Gender: Male
Sign: Gemini

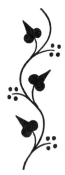

Bayberry

Candleberry, waxberry, wax myrtle

Bayberry is a dense evergreen, two to four feet high, with gray outer and reddish-brown inner bark. It has dark green leaves, dotted on both sides, and bluish-white berries. It is very fragrant.

Parts used: Bark, berries

Therapeutic Profile

Stimulant
Astringent
Diaphoretic
Expectorant
Tonic
Antibiotic

Recent Research

One component in bayberry, myricitrin, has been shown to be toxic to bacteria and parasites. Studies also show it relieves fevers.

Medicinal Uses; Catalysts and Combinations

Bayberry has been considered one of the most important herbs in botanical medicine, but its use must be restricted. It is an excellent liver tonic, and is useful in treating diarrhea. It has been used to cleanse mucous membranes and restore them to normal. It makes an effective gargle for a sore throat, and may be used as a douche to treat vaginal infections. When the berries are boiled, they form a waxy substance that can then be used as a poultice for hemorrhoids or external ulcers. Taken in large doses it will induce vomiting and can cause a severe drop in blood pressure. It combines well with ginger and cayenne for colds and fevers.

Dosage and Administration

Steep 1 teaspoon of bark in 1 cup of boiling water. If the bark is powdered, use 1–4 grams, or use 10–20 drops of the tincture.

Gathering and Useful Notes

Gather roots in early spring or late autumn and peel bark before drying. For decoction, use 1 ounce to 1 pint of water; use as a douche or gargle. The powder may be used as a sniff for sinus congestion. Use no longer than 4 days. Side effects may include nausea or vomiting.

History and Lore

Bayberry has been used in folk practices to attract money, and bayberry candles were often burned for this purpose. The wax is easily removed from the berries by boiling them in water, wherein it floats to the top. Its aromatic properties have made it a popular candle at Christmastime. It is common to swamps and marshes and one American Indian tribe, the Louisiana Choctaws, employed it as a fever remedy. The white settlers discovered its use for dysentery and it became a very popular herb for the next 200 years. It is now often used as an insecticide.

Correspondences

Planet: Mercury
Element: Air
Gender: Male
Sign: Virgo

Bilberry

Blueberry, dyeberry, huckleberry

Bilberry is a perennial shrub, common to Europe and North America. It grows one to one-and-a-half feet high, with an angular green stem that is branched. It has alternate leaves that are dark green and shiny, with red, pink, and white flowers and blue-black berries.

Parts used: Berry and leaf

Therapeutic Profile

Antiseptic

Antioxidant

Anti-inflammatory

Astringent

Diuretic

Tonic

Recent Research

Clinical tests show positive results in visual disfunctions and disorders. Bilberry is an antioxidant that prevents free radical damage in human tissue. It has antiviral properties in cell cultures for herpes and influenza.

Medicinal Uses; Catalysts and Combinations

Taken consistently, bilberry helps build better vision caused by weak capillaries. It is good for night blindness and any kind of arterial weakness. Bilberry has been used medicinally in the treatment of diarrhea and urinary disorders. It helps regulate blood sugar levels and is a nutritive tonic for wasting diseases. It is recommended for use during pregnancy, and helps prevent varicose veins. Certain chemicals in bilberry are very active free radical scavengers, and it may prove useful against cancer. It is effective in repairing bruises.

Diabetics should use it under the guidance of a health-care professional. It combines well with goldenseal and fenugreek.

Dosage and Administration

Boil 1 teaspoon of the dried berries in 1 cup of water. Drink 1–2 cups a day. Capsules can be used with the dry extract, up to 480 milligrams daily.

Gathering and Useful Notes

Gather berries when plant is fully developed but before berries are ripe, usually between July and September. To make an extract for the treatment of viruses, use ⅓ ounce dried berries in 1 cup of water; let stand for 8 hours.

History and Lore

Bilberry is part of the blueberry family and has been associated with protection in folklore. Blueberry pies were eaten to protect one from psychic attack, and blueberries were placed on doorways to fend off evil. As a phytomedicine, bilberry has enjoyed wide popularity in Europe for protection against eye diseases and peripheral vascular disorders. It has aroused interest as a therapeutic agent in the U.S. since World War II, when it was determined that Allied pilots had better eyesight in twilight than the enemy. Since bilberry jam was part of their diet, it was believed that this may have been the cause of their heightened vision. Thus began the first among many studies on bilberry's effectiveness.

Correspondences

  Planet: Moon
  Element: Water
  Gender: Female
  Sign: Cancer

Black Cohosh

Black snake root, squaw root, rattleweed

Cohosh is native to North America, tending to prefer higher elevations. It has a large knotty rootstock and a stem that grows up to eight to nine feet high. The leaves are oblong and saw-toothed, often splitting into three divisions; the flowers are very small and white.

Part used: Root

Therapeutic Profile

Antispasmodic
Anti-inflammatory
Emmenagogue
Diuretic
Nervine

Recent Research

Clinical findings validate black cohosh's uterine contractile activity, and there is also evidence for its hypotensive and anti-inflammatory properties. It has been shown to relieve hot flashes in controlled studies and, in some cases, vaginal atrophy. It is now being investigated for cholesterol regulation.

Medicinal Uses; Catalysts and Combinations

Black cohosh is one of the estrogenic herbs now called "phytoestrogens," which means it is capable of exerting effects similar to estrogen but without its negative side effects. It is a uterine tonic for menstrual abnormalities and also lessens the symptoms of menopause—in Germany, more than one million women have used it with great success. It is active in the treatment of bronchitis, cough, and chorea, as well as rheumatic conditions and neurological pain, such as sciatica. It reduces spasms of any kind and it is a relaxing nervine. However, in some people it may cause heart palpitations. It is good combined with valerian and hops for nerves and vitex for menopause.

Dosage and Administration

Boil 2 teaspoons of the root in 1 pint of water. Take 2–3 tablespoons up to 6 times daily. As a tincture, take 10–60 drops. Commercial capsules are popular for menopause and PMS complaints. .

Gathering and Useful Notes

The seed produces root during the winter and emerges the following spring. Collect rootstock the next fall, after leaves have dried somewhat. The roots should be cut lengthwise and dried slowly. It should also be boiled slowly, at least ½ hour, and then stored in a closed container. Drink cold.

History and Lore

In folklore, black cohosh has been associated with love, courage, and protection. It was often used to invoke Venusian qualities, and was placed in love sachets. Long known among the American Indians as a treatment for uterine disorders, black cohosh was one of the earliest herbs introduced to American medicine by the early settlers. It was called squaw root. Cohosh was one of the principle ingredients in the first menopausal compound, created by a Miss Lydia Pinkham in 1876, and it made her quite famous. Today it must be ecologically harvested, as its popularity has caused it to become endangered.

Correspondences

Planet: Venus
Element: Air
Gender: Female
Sign: Libra

Blessed Thistle

Holy thistle, blessed cardus, bitter thistle

The plant is an annual with an erect, branched stem and thin, hairy leaves two to three inches long and lance-shaped. Its flowers are yellow, sitting on the end of the branches, and it has long, cylindrical seeds.

Parts used: Leaves, flowery twigs, seeds

Therapeutic Profile

Antibiotic
Bitter
Galactagogue
Febrifuge
Expectorant
Diaphoretic

Recent Research

The herb has demonstrated antitumor activity in mice experiments, and antibacterial activity against a number of organisms. It has anti-yeast properties in vitro, especially against candida.

Medicinal Uses; Catalysts and Combinations

Blessed thistle has principally been used to treat appetite loss (anorexia) and indigestion. It is good for liver congestion and related symptoms, such as jaundice and hepatitis. Use it to bring down fevers and lessen mucus congestion. It is excellent for cleansing, since it causes perspiration, and may also be used to treat diarrhea. It is sometimes combined with black cohosh and cramp bark to correct hormonal imbalances that lead to irregular menstrual cycles. It is also useful to stop bleeding or resolve blood clots. For stimulation of mother's milk, use with raspberry and marshmallow.

Dosage and Administration

Pour 1 cup of boiling water over leaves and let steep 10 minutes. It may be drunk 2–3 times daily. In tincture form, take 10–20 drops; or take 1–3 capsules a day.

Gathering and Useful Notes

The leaves and flowers should be collected while still in bloom, usually before August, and dried in the shade. Sometimes the plant will regenerate, making a second cutting possible. Seeds are gathered in the fall. When making an infusion for nursing mothers, it should be made cold and steeped several hours.

History and Lore

Blessed thistle was a favorite in folklore for protection against hexes. It was associated with Pan in Greek mythology and therefore became associated with sexuality. In astrology, it was attributed to Pluto, which is associated with procreation, regeneration, and also with the relationships of generations; that is, with cultural preservation. European monks used it as a cure for smallpox. It is still thought of in many places as an aphrodisiac.

Correspondences

Planet: Pluto
Element: Water
Gender: Male
Sign: Scorpio

Bloodroot

King root, redroot, sweet slumber

The herb is a small perennial, around six inches high, with roots about finger size that exude red juice when cut; after it is dried, the root is yellow. It has basal, veined leaves stemming from buds on the roots, with white flowers.

Part used: Root

Therapeutic Profile

Cardiac
Pectoral
Stimulant
Expectorant
Antiseptic

Recent Research

It has been demonstrated that bloodroot is a poisonous narcotic and it is included on the FDA's unsafe herb list. However, topically it has been shown to be helpful in relieving eczema, and recent studies indicate it helps prevent cavities.

Medicinal Uses; Catalysts and Combinations

Bloodroot has been traditionally used as an expectorant for coughs, asthma, or sinus congestion. In older herbals, it is one of the favorite remedies for bronchitis. It was often used in cough syrups with cherry bark or eucalyptus for flavoring. It can be applied externally to treat skin diseases, such as athlete's foot, fungus, and burns. It acts as stimulation for poor circulation. It may be combined with lobelia for asthma or cayenne for pharyngitis. Large doses are dangerous and may be fatal.

Dosage and Administration

Put 1 teaspoon root in 1 cup water, bring to boil, and steep for 10–15 minutes. Drink 1–2 times daily.

Gathering and Useful Notes

Dig the roots in early summer or after the leaves have dried in late fall. Dry carefully in the shade. It may be stored to use as a gargle if a large infusion is made. The powder can be applied directly to the skin or a compress can be made by soaking the powder in cold water for 12 hours, and then bringing to a boil; when cool enough, pour onto a towel and apply to the skin.

History and Lore

Bloodroot was thought to protect the home; the best kind to use were the reddest. The root was worn to avert negativity. It was also called "sweet slumber" because of its deadly character; taken in large quantities, it is quite poisonous. Although this aspect of the herb was well respected, it was nonetheless used by many American Indian tribes as a remedy for rheumatism, ringworm, sore throat, and skin ulcers. Its Mars-like character is demonstrated by the fact that its red juice was used as a facial dye for war paint.

Correspondences

   Planet: Mars
   Element: Fire
   Gender: Male
   Sign: Aries

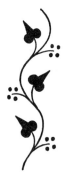

Boneset

Crosswort, feverwort, Indian sage

Boneset is a perennial common to swamp areas with a rough, hairy stem that reaches one to five inches high. The root grows horizontal and crooked, and the leaves are serrated and pointed. It has white blossoms and bitter fruit.

Parts used: All of the dried herb above ground

Therapeutic Profile

Bitter
Diaphoretic
Emetic
Tonic
Laxative
Febrifuge

Recent Research

The leaves contain an ingredient that destroys parasites and worms. Studies have found it to be a useful appetite stimulant and new research indicates it may have antitumor properties.

Medicinal Uses; Catalysts and Combinations

The herb is best used for treatment of influenza. Boneset is a relaxing herb for muscles, stomach, bowel, and uterus. It therefore is excellent for aches and pains due to flu, as well as rheumatism or arthritis. It promotes perspiration and is good for treating fevers. It is particularly helpful in relieving mucus congestion. It is effective as a laxative and aids in the secretion of bile. It has been used to treat jaundice and skin diseases. For treatment of flu, combine with yarrow, cayenne, or ginger.

Dosage and Administration

Use 1 teaspoon of the herb in 1 cup of water; bring to a boil, steep 20 minutes, and strain. Take 3–6 times daily. As a tincture, take 10–40 drops at a time.

Gathering and Useful Notes

Gather as soon as flowers open in late summer or early fall. If taken as a tea, it should be drunk as hot as possible and very frequently if treating a fever. Capsules are not as effective and often need to be taken in large quantities, up to 30 a day. It is a very safe herb.

History and Lore

In folklore, boneset was thought to fend off evil spirits, and was used in exorcisms. It was popular among American settlers at least 100 years before being listed in any compiled pharmacological text. It was a favorite among the American Indians for fevers and colds. Its name is said to come from an influenza so rampant and wretched that it seemed to cause its sufferers to feel like all their bones were broken; boneset was successful in treating this flu.

Correspondences

Planet: Saturn
Element: Water
Gender: Female
Sign: Capricorn

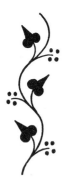

Buchu
Oval buchu, bookoo

Buchu is small shrub, growing two to three feet high, common to South America. It has glossy pale-green leaves with strongly curved tips and serrated margins. It has white-pinkish petals and small capsule-like fruit.

Part used: Leaves

Therapeutic Profile
Antiseptic
Astringent
Diuretic
Diaphoretic

Recent Research
Its efficacy in treating urinary tract infections has been found to be due to its volatile oil, which is called buchu camphor or diosphenol. It is used in some proprietary drugs as a urinary antiseptic.

Medicinal Uses; Catalysts and Combinations
Buchu is one of the best-known diuretics and is excellent for kidney disorders or any infection of the genito-urinary system. It alleviates a high-acid urine and it is a good tonic for the prostate or for prostate enlargement, especially if treated early. It may be effective in the early treatment of diabetes and is a component in some fever remedies. Complementary agents include uva ursi, alfalfa, and juniper.

Dosage and Administration

Use 1 tablespoon of dried leaves in 1 cup of water; steep 20 minutes. Take 4 tablespoons 3–4 times a day. As a tincture, take 10-20 drops 3 times daily.

Gathering and Useful Notes

Leaves should be collected when the plant is flowering or bearing fruit. It works best if taken as a cold-water infusion. Do not boil, as this dissipates the most active ingredient, its volatile oil.

History and Lore

In some cultures, buchu was a favorite herb for use in divination. It was believed that one acquired psychic powers when drinking the tea. It was also used to produce dreams if burned as an incense in the bedroom. In 1847, Mr. Henry Helmbold became known as the Buchu King because he made a fortune selling his buchu compound. It made him so famous he even aspired to be president of the United States. Buchu has been used for many centuries in Africa, originally utilized by the Hottentots (bookoo is a Hottentot word).

Correspondences

Planet: Moon
Element: Water
Gender: Female
Sign: Cancer

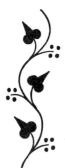

Burdock

Beggar's buttons, cocklebur, happy major

Burdock is a common plant in the U.S. and Europe, growing along fences, walls, and roadsides. It has a long fleshy gray root with a reddish stem and woolly branches. The leaves are oblong, green, and hairy; the flowers appear in loose purple clusters.

Parts used: Root, seed, leaves

Therapeutic Profile

Diaphoretic
Antibiotic
Alternative
Cholagogue
Hepatic
Diuretic

Recent Research

At least fourteen compounds have been identified in the root that possess antibacterial and antifungal properties. It has been shown to reduce tumors in mice. Studies have demonstrated that it is a therapeutic agent in bile secretion and it is being investigated for its hypoglycemic action.

Medicinal Uses; Catalysts and Combinations

Burdock is excellent in neutralizing and eliminating poisons from the system and it is therefore part of many detoxification programs. As a tea, it has been used for stomach complaints. It aids digestion and appetite. Both seeds and leaves are good for treating skin disorders, especially psoriasis. It is effective for arthritis, sciatica, and rheumatism. Burdock is especially rich in minerals and has long been used as a strong blood builder. It can also lower blood sugar. It promotes good kidney function and has a cooling effect on the body, thus aiding in fever reduction. It combines well with red clover and cleavers.

Dosage and Administration

Place 1 teaspoon of the chopped root in 1½ cups of water; bring to a boil and simmer 10–15 minutes. Drink 2–3 times daily. In extract form, take 10–25 drops daily. Capsules may be taken 1–3 times a day.

Gathering and Useful Notes

Collect roots in spring or fall, when the plant is two years old. Use seeds with more caution than the rest of the plant. Leaves are best used for stimulation of bile secretion. As a hot compress, pour burdock tea over a towel and apply externally as needed for sores or bites.

History and Lore

The name "burdock" is a combination of "bur," for its spiked seed covers, and "dock," which simply means "plant." In some cultures, burdock roots were collected, strung on red thread, and worn for protection. It was gathered during the waning moon. The burdock burrs have been the playthings of children wherever they grow and are referred to in Shakespeare's *King Lear*. It has been listed for centuries in numerous pharmacological texts in many countries. American Indians used it for 200 years in treating pain in the joints. The Chinese use the herb for its calming effects. The herbalist Hildegard of Bingen used burdock to treat tumors. Recently it has been investigated by biotechnologists to introduce cancer-preventive chemicals into common foods.

Correspondences

Planet: Venus
Element: Water
Gender: Female
Sign: Libra

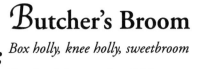

Butcher's Broom

Box holly, knee holly, sweetbroom

Butcher's broom is a fairly common, short, evergreen shrub that grows throughout the Mediterranean. It has stiff, leaf-like twigs, clustered principally around the top.

Parts used: Root, leaves

Therapeutic Profile

Anti-inflammatory
Diuretic
Aperient
Diaphoretic

Recent Research

Investigations in France indicate that an extract of butcher's broom produces vasoconstriction; early trials in humans point to its effectiveness in venous disorders. It has demonstrated anti-inflammatory properties. The saponins from the plant are the basis of many steroid drugs.

Medicinal Uses; Catalysts and Combinations

The herb straightens weak blood vessels and discourages the formation of clots. Its primary use is as an antithrombosis agent in cases of phlebitis and arteriosclerosis. It is also good for varicose veins and hemorrhoids. It has been used to facilitate cellulite reduction and is good for leg cramps. It is an excellent blood purifier and is good for jaundice and gout. Complementary agents include ginkgo, ginger, and bilberry.

Dosage and Administration

Simmer ½ ounce of dried leaves in 1 pint of water for 20 minutes. Take 1–3 times daily. Capsules can be taken up to three times a day, or take 10–20 drops of the extract in water or juice.

Gathering and Useful Notes

Butcher's broom is frequently confused with a similar variety of common roadside shrubs, often called "broom," which grow in the U.S., not in the Mediterranean. Because of its steroid properties, butcher's broom is good when used as an ointment for leg pain or hemorrhoids. If taken orally, it may cause stomach upset; if so, cut back the dosage.

History and Lore

In folklore it was believed that ritual use of butcher's broom involved making an infusion and sprinkling it around a home to rid it of ghosts. It was also thought to invoke spirits of the air when thrown to the winds from a hilltop. As early as the first century, it was recommended by the healer Dioscorides as a cleanser. The seventeenth-century astrologer Nicholas Culpepper, who wrote the first herbal in English, believed it could heal broken bones. There is a legend that the Virgin Mary was startled at the plant on the flight into Egypt because it made a loud noise as they passed by.

Correspondences

    Planet: Uranus
    Element: Air
    Gender: Male
    Sign: Aquarius

Cascara Sagrada

Sacred bark, California buckthorn, chittem bark

Cascara is a deciduous tree common to the mountain regions of North America. It grows about twenty feet high and has reddish brown bark, often covered with gray lichen patches. It has elliptical saw-toothed leaves that are two to six inches long, large clusters of greenish flowers, and pea-sized berries.

Part used: Bark

Therapeutic Profile

Laxative
Bitter
Hepatic

Recent Research

Extracts of Cascara sagrada have been shown to have antiviral activity against herpes simplex II, as well as antileukemic properties in cell cultures. It has been demonstrated to have antibacterial action in the intestines and one study showed it has chelative agents to prevent the formation of kidney stones.

Medicinal Uses; Catalysts and Combinations

This herb is one of the best plant laxatives, encouraging bowel movement in a non-habit forming action. It is also a bitter tonic for the liver and gallbladder. It is good for flatulence and is effective in the treatment of jaundice, enlarged liver, colitis, and hemorrhoids. It combines well with senna, aloe, and beet root.

Dosage and Administration

As a tea, drink 1–2 cups before meals or before bedtime. Or it may be taken in a fluid tincture, 20-25 drops, 2–3 times a day until desired effects are achieved. It is also included in commercial preparations in capsule form; take as directed.

Gathering and Useful Notes

The bark should be gathered and dried for at least a year before use. The longer it is aged, the milder the cathartic action. It tends to cause griping if harvested too soon. It is best to steep 1 teaspoon of the bark in 1 cup of water for 1 hour before drinking. Do not take over an extended period of time. Do not take if you are pregnant or have an ulcer.

History and Lore

In folklore, the herb was thought to be associated with money and good luck. If an infusion was sprinkled around the home before going to court, it was helpful in winning the court case. It is believed that the early Spanish priests of the Pacific Northwest learned of this "sacred bark" from the California Indian natives, and it soon became the most famous laxative in the known world. It is the foundation for all natural cleansing programs. Dr. Christopher believed that when the colon is clean, we are able to fight disease much easier, for health begins in the bowel: "When we are free from toxins in the eliminative system, then the whole body can be fed properly, and we begin to live!" (*School for Natural Healing*, p. 196).

Correspondences

   Planet: Mercury
   Element: Air
   Gender: Male
   Sign: Gemini

Catnip

Catmint, field balm, catswort

Like all species of the mint family, catnip has a square stem; it is hairy and grows about two to four feet high. It has oblong pointed leaves and white or mauve flowers that are slightly aromatic.

Parts used: Leaves, flowers

Therapeutic Profile

Carminative
Antispasmodic
Diaphoretic
Sedative

Recent Research

An extract of catnip has been found to be toxic to cancer cells in vitro. Preliminary research shows it may have antibiotic properties. It has been shown to be high in iron and is therefore efficacious in treating anemia.

Medicinal Uses; Catalysts and Combinations

Catnip has traditionally been used in the treatment of colds and flu, and it will also bring down fevers. It is good for digestive problems and appears to kill bacteria in the intestinal tract. It has been used to treat colic in infants and has a calming effect that is safe for children as well as adults. It is useful in treating insomnia, anemia, and nervousness. Complementary agents include ginger and peppermint for nervous stomach, and cayenne for colds.

Dosage and Administration

Pour 1 cup of boiling water over 2 teaspoons of the dried herb and steep 10 minutes. It may be drunk several times a day. Or take the tincture, using 1 teaspoon 2–3 times daily.

Gathering and Useful Notes

The leaves and flowering tops should be collected during the summer. It likes full sun. It can be cut back and harvested twice the same year. An infusion can be made from the flowers and used as an enema for nervousness and headache for speedy relief. Steep, do not boil.

History and Lore

Catnip originally was used in Siberia and the High Himalayas, and eventually migrated to Europe and North America. Large catnip leaves were often used as bookmarks in medieval texts. American Indians used the tea for childhood colic and eventually it became so famous for digestive complaints that today it is often referred to as "Nature's Alka Seltzer." Because of its delightful influence on cats, it was believed to create a psychic bond between cats and their owners. It was used in love sachets and, when hung over a doorway, was thought to attract harmony.

Correspondences

Planet: Venus
Element: Water
Gender: Female
Sign: Taurus

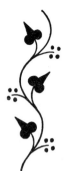

Cat's Claw

Uncaria, uña de gato

Cat's claw is a large, woody vine, as long as 100 feet in length, found at high elevations in the Peruvian rainforests. The vines have yellow-white, bell-shaped flowers and cat claw-like thorns that grow on trees to which it can attach itself.

Parts used: Bark and root; roots are now protected

Therapeutic Profile

Adaptogen
Antioxidant
Antibiotic
Immunostimulant
Anti-inflammatory
Antitumor
Laxative

Recent Research

Worldwide research is being conducted exploring the use of cat's claw in the treatment of cancer and AIDS. The triterpenes in the herb boost T cell activity. Peruvian doctors have been using it in the treatment of fourteen kinds of cancer, and at least two compounds have been isolated for use in controlling viruses.

Medicinal Uses; Catalysts and Combinations

Therapeutic applications for cat's claw abound and are growing as research continues to expand in this area. It has impressive anti-inflammatory properties, making it an excellent tonic for arthritis and fibromyalgia. It promotes colonic health but may give some people diarrhea. The alkaloids in the herb appear to target the immune system, the intestinal tract, and the cardiovascular system most effectively. It is a very powerful antioxidant. Peruvian women use it to recover from childbirth. Herbal extracts should be blended with the whole herb for greatest efficacy. It can be combined with Pau d'Arco and echinacea.

Dosage and Administration

Use 1 teaspoon of dried bark per cup, simmer 10–15 minutes, and drink 1–2 cups daily for antioxidant protection. The tea is extremely bitter, however, so most prefer to take the herb in capsule form, 1–3 grams daily. Therapeutic doses range from 3–20 grams daily, used under the care of a health-care professional.

Gathering and Useful Notes

The bark is harvested and stripped; only the inner bark and root are used to make a decoction. If bought commercially, cat's claw must contain "Uncaria tomentosa" in order to be effective. Not all that is labeled "cat's claw" has this essential component. Do not use if pregnant or nursing or if you have a transplanted organ. The herb may cause a change in stool consistency.

History and Lore

The native Indian tribes of Peru believed cat's claw was a sacred herb because of its seemingly unlimited therapeutic qualities. Its Latin name, *uncaria*, is from the root *uncus*, which means "hook" (since its thorns resemble the claws of a cat). Although botanical references to the herb date as far back as the 1700s, it was only rediscovered in 1974 by a European scientist after a journalist traveling to Peru gave it to a relative who had cancer and was cured. It gained such great interest around the world that studies in at least seven clinics have conducted research on the herb in the past fifteen years. It is believed that cat's claw was one of the principle herbs used by indigenous Amazon shamans.

Correspondences

   Planet: Uranus
   Element: Air
   Gender: Male
   Sign: Aquarius

Cayenne

Capsicum, chili, bird pepper

Cayenne is a perennial that grows in most tropical areas, and an annual outside the tropics. It grows up to three feet high, and has a woody stem, which branches near the top. It has ovate leaves and drooping white flowers. The fruit is a many-seeded red pod.

Part used: Fruit

Therapeutic Profile

Stimulant
Antibiotic
Antioxidant
Cardiotonic
Decongestant
Carminative
Antiseptic
Hemostatic
Rubefacient

Recent Research

Research has demonstrated that sensory nerve endings become insensitive to pain in areas treated with capsicum. It also appears to protect lungs from free radical damage due to some chemicals. It lowers cholesterol in clinical studies.

Medicinal Uses; Catalysts and Combinations

Cayenne is most known for its use as a systemic stimulant, acting to strengthen the heart, arteries, and nerves. It is an excellent tonic for digestion and will generally cure ulcers or gastritis. It is used for colds, flu, and as a gargle for laryngitis. It neutralizes blood pressure and is a warming agent for arthritis or muscle pain. Capsicum balms are useful for fibromyalgia and diuretic neuropathic pain as well. It is used to fight most any kind of infection, and is effective in stimulating the appetite. It combines well with garlic and echinacea as an infection fighter and with gotu kola as a stimulant.

Dosage and Administration
Use ½ to 1 teaspoon of dried pepper in 1 cup of hot water and drink warm. It may be taken in capsule form 1–3 times a day, if drinking it proves too hot to the taste. Sprinkle freely on foods.

Gathering and Useful Notes
The fruit should be gathered when it is fully ripe and it should be dried upside down in the shade. Be sure and harvest before the first frost. Cayenne makes a good ointment for muscle or joint pain; however, prolonged application to the skin may cause blisters. Never apply to mucous membranes. Excessive consumption may cause kidney problems. A hot compress can be made by pouring hot tea over a towel and applying directly to the skin.

History and Lore
Members of the genus *Capsicum* are native to the Western hemisphere and were misnamed "pepper" by the Spanish explorers when they first encountered the herb, thinking it was the peppercorn of India. They brought the herb back to Europe, where it quickly gained wide popularity. In some places, red peppers are carried in amulets for protection. In Mexico, a branch was brushed against a sick person and then buried, to carry away the illness. There is a legend that if someone happens to die on the prairie, the vultures will not touch the body if the person had eaten a lot of cayenne. In the West Indies it was so popular that the natives had no fear of yellow fever as long as they carried the herb. The name is from the Greek *kapto*, "I bite," and it is often called the biting plant. It is a favorite food of the Hunza.

Correspondences
Planet: Mars
Element: Fire
Gender: Male
Sign: Aries

Chamomile

Roman chamomile, German chamomile

Roman chamomile is a low-growing perennial with a stem that trails the ground without rooting. It has alternate, dissected leaves and solitary flowerheads eight to ten inches high that are yellow and white. German chamomile is an annual, similar in appearance and native to Europe.

Part used: Flowers

Therapeutic Profile

Antispasmodic
Anti-inflammatory
Carminative
Vulnerary
Nervine

Recent Research

Recent studies indicate that chamomile works as a uterine tonic. Studies indicate it possesses antibacterial and anti-inflammatory properties. It shows promise as a chemopreventive agent.

Medicinal Uses; Catalysts and Combinations

Chamomile is most often used as a remedy for nerves and insomnia. It is safe enough to use with children. It is also a good antispasmodic and is useful for menstrual cramps and backaches. It has been used as a gastrointestinal tonic and is particularly helpful for flatulence. It makes a good mouthwash and also a wash for sore eyes. Externally it is useful for speeding the healing of wounds. A hot, soaked towel of the infusion can relieve earache pain. Complementary agents include valerian and hops for stress; lobelia for earaches; and peppermint for digestion.

Dosage and Administration

Pour 1 cup of boiling water over 2 teaspoons of the dried flowers and steep for 5 minutes. Drink with meals. An extract of 10–20 drops may be taken once or twice a day.

Gathering and Useful Notes

Flowers are gathered all summer when they are open on the plant. Do not collect in the morning when wet with dew. Dry at low temperatures. The compress for cramps may be made by soaking a hot towel in the tea and applying it hot. Some people have shown allergic reactions to chamomile. Do not take for prolonged periods of time.

History and Lore

In folklore it was believed that if chamomile were planted in a garden, it will be the guardian spirit for whatever else was planted there. It was said to guarantee the success of any intention when included in an amulet. It has long enjoyed great popularity in Europe. It was also used as a sleep and meditation incense. A famous old saying went, "How the Doctor's brow should smile, crowned with wreaths of chamomile." Chamomile is still an immensely popular herb in both the U.S. and in Europe, and 4,000 tons of it are grown and harvested annually. It has long been a popular hair rinse; not as a dye, but as a brightener.

Correspondences

Planet: Sun
Element: Fire
Gender: Male
Sign: Leo

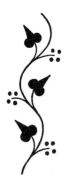

Chaparral

Greesewood, creosote bush, black bush

Chaparral is a leafy evergreen shrub with small, olive-green resinous leaves, bright yellow flowers, and a small, white, woolly seed pod. It is native to the American Southwest and Mexico.

Parts used: Leaves, stems

Therapeutic Profile

Antibiotic
Antioxidant
Antiseptic
Alternative
Expectorant

Recent Research

Chaparral is being investigated for its use as a lymph cleanser in the treatment of cancer and leukemia. It contains a powerful antioxidant known as NDGA (nordihydroguairetic acid). In animal studies, it slows the aging process.

Medicinal Uses; Catalysts and Combinations

Chaparral is a powerful herbal antibiotic, effective against bacteria, viruses, and parasites. It is a herbal antioxidant but should not be used frequently as a defense in the way that most antioxidants are used, because taken in large quantities it is poisonous. However, combined with other herbs, it can be very effective in rebuilding the body from major diseases such as cancer. It is a blood purifier, and may be taken in small quantities for its vasodepressant effects, or for rheumatic pains. Externally it makes a good poultice for wounds. Use with red clover, dandelion, echinacea, and astragalus for serious diseases.

Dosage and Administration

Pour boiling water over ½ ounce of dried leaves and steep 10–15 minutes. Or take 10–30 drops of the tincture.

Gathering and Useful Notes

Gather when the seeds are mature in early fall. Dry slowly and carefully to preserve the volatile oils. Make a liniment by steeping leaves in rubbing alcohol and applying directly to the skin. Long-term use has caused liver damage and it is labeled dangerous by the FDA. Use only with the guidance of a health-care professional.

History and Lore

The herb has a long history of use by Native Americans despite the caution in its use today. The Indians used it as a remedy for cancer and arthritis. Over time, it has been used as a cure for almost everything, including as a hair tonic. A number of studies have been done in this century with chaparral, and mysteries still surround it. Although it is toxic in large amounts in healthy people, it cures tumors and skin cancers in some subjects. When mosquitoes were fed the compound NDGA, their lifespan lengthened from twenty-nine to forty-five days. The implications of this kind of research are rather remarkable. One of its names, "creosote bush," is derived from the name of the oil, which is used to treat wood. This perennial bush has been carbon-dated to be 13,000 years old.

Correspondences

Planet: Mercury
Element: Earth
Gender: Female
Sign: Virgo

Chickweed

Satin flower, starweed, winterweed

Chickweed is a common herb growing along roadsides around the world. It has creeping brittle stems, four to ten inches long, and ovate leaves, with tiny white flowers that bloom continuously.

Parts used: All of the herb above ground

Therapeutic Profile

Antibiotic
Emollient
Nutritive
Vulnerary
Laxative

Recent Research

Modern research has demonstrated that chickweed has antibiotic properties. It appears to be effective against certain respiratory pathogens, and it has a very high nutritive content.

Medicinal Uses; Catalysts and Combinations

Chickweed is a mild laxative when ingested, and it is often drunk as a tea for rheumatic pains. It supports the gastrointestinal tract and is one of the most nutritious foods in the herbal kingdom. Externally, it is more commonly used as a salve for skin rashes, psoriasis, or eczema. It is good applied to cuts and wounds. It combines well with marshmallow as an ointment, as well as chaparral for drawing out poisons. It is sometimes added to formulas for weight reduction, since it is such a concentrated, fat-free food source.

Dosage and Administration

Use 1 ounce of the dried herb in 1 cup of boiling water, and steep 5 minutes. Drink 3 times a day. Or take 1 teaspoon of the extract twice a day.

Gathering and Useful Notes

Chickweed can be gathered year round, wherever it grows. It can be eaten as a vegetable, like any cooked green. Medicinally, it is best used externally. Use the fresh leaves with a Vaseline base for an ointment. A strong infusion can be made and poured into the bath for skin diseases, or made into a salve.

History and Lore

In folklore, chickweed was used to attract a lover. It was also believed that once gained, one's true love would remain faithful if blessed by the spirit of the herb. It was associated with the moon and dreaming. The Iroquois used the herb as a poultice for wounds. The herbalist Dr. John Christopher made a famous salve called "black healing ointment" with chickweed as a base, which cured many complaints of the skin, including skin cancer. There is an old custom of giving chickweed seed to birds. It is also believed to break down cellulite.

Correspondences

   Planet: Moon
   Element: Water
   Gender: Female
   Sign: Cancer

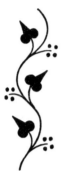

Cleavers

Bedstraw, coachweed, goose grass

Cleavers is an annual herb growing in moist places, usually along riverbanks. It has a slight, square stem that is two to four feet high with rough linear leaves wrapping around it in whorls. It has greenish-white or white flowers that bloom all summer and a small globular fruit with one seed.

Parts used: All of the herb above ground

Therapeutic Profile

Diuretic
Alternative
Astringent
Tonic
Diaphoretic
Antibiotic
Hepatic
Nutritive

Recent Research

Some studies indicate that the herb has antibiotic properties. There is research in the use of cleavers for its hypotensive activity.

Medicinal Uses; Catalysts and Combinations

Cleavers is an excellent tonic for the lymph system and one of the most effective blood purifiers in the herbal kingdom. It is useful in treating swollen glands, tonsillitis, and urinary tract infections. Its diuretic properties help relieve bloating and excess weight. It is very astringent and makes an excellent wash for the face. It is a general tonic for the liver, kidney, and pancreas, and helps rid the system of toxic wastes. It is best combined with uva ursi, buchu, and marshmallow for the treatment of urinary tract infections, and echinacea for lymphatic infections.

Dosage and Administration

Pour 1 cup of boiling water over 2–3 teaspoons of the dried herb, and steep 10 minutes. Drink several times a day. It can be taken in capsule form, up to 15 a day, or applied locally as needed.

Gathering and Useful Notes

Cleavers should be gathered before it flowers, from June through September, and then dried in the shade. A wash can be made from the infusion for sunburn and freckles. Make the salve by mixing fresh-squeezed juice with butter or Vaseline; apply topically every 3 hours.

History and Lore

Cleavers was often called "fragrant bedstraw" and was worn to attract love. It was also believed to protect one from snakes. The Swiss used the seeds as a coffee substitute. For a long time it was thought to be particularly good for any kind of water diseases, such as dropsy, which today we call edema. It also makes an excellent vegetable.

Correspondences

Planet: Moon
Element: Water
Gender: Female
Sign: Cancer

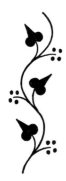

Clove

Mother cloves, girofle

Cloves grow on an evergreen tree about thirty feet high, with extensive branches, yellow bark, and rose-colored, bell-shaped flowers. It has ovate leaves around five inches long. The flower buds are the cloves when dried, which are about three-fourths inches long and dark brown.

Part used: Flower buds

Therapeutic Profile

Stimulant
Carminative
Antiseptic
Rubefacient
Vermifuge
Anti-inflammatory

Recent Research

The oil has been shown to have anti-inflammatory properties in both animals and humans. The extract is useful in suppressing plaque in studies, and it has strong antibacterial activity.

Medicinal Uses; Catalysts and Combinations

Clove has been valued as a powerful carminative; its aromatic properties promote digestion and relieve nausea. It can help stop vomiting. Clove oil is good for the pain of toothache when applied directly to a cavity. Some dentists use it as an oral antiseptic and as a disinfectant for root canals. It is a useful treatment for diarrhea, intestinal worms, and parasites. It stimulates the circulatory system and strengthens the liver. Combine with cinnamon and spearmint for nausea.

Dosage and Administration
Pour 1 pint of boiling water over 1 teaspoon cloves and steep 20 minutes. Or put a few drops in water and drink for nausea. Use oil directly on the tooth for pain.

Gathering and Useful Notes
Trees do not yield their flowers for at least six years. The flower buds should be gathered just before they ripen, at the pink stage. Buds are often caught on outstretched blankets laid on the ground. Dry quickly. Cloves are particularly helpful for vomiting and nausea during pregnancy.

History and Lore
The principal place where cloves grow is in Tanzania, which produces at least 75 percent of the world's supply. It has a history in China, where it is famous for disguising bad breath. Those who spoke to the Emperor were required to eat cloves before the visit. Europeans imported it as a preservative for food and discovered its value as a spice. Pomanders made with cloves were made as a bug repellent and to cover decayed odors caused by lack of refrigeration. It was believed that to inhale clove would stave melancholy. Clove has long been thought to be an aphrodisiac.

Correspondences
  Planet: Venus
  Element: Earth
  Gender: Female
  Sign: Taurus

Comfrey

Blackwort, healing herb, knitbone

Comfrey is a perennial that likes meadows. It has a hairy, hollow stem and large ovate leaves, larger at the bottom and tongue shaped. The root is black and deeply wrinkled, with white glutinous juice. The pale white or lavender flowers are long and hollow and terminate at the many branches; the seeds are small and black.

Parts used: Root, leaves

Therapeutic Profile

Demulcent
Astringent
Expectorant
Vulnerary
Pectoral
Hemostatic
Anti-inflammatory
Nutritive

Recent Research

Comfrey contains allantoin, which has been identified as an agent that stimulates new cell growth or cell proliferation. This makes it useful for wound healing, but findings indicate that certain alkaloids taken in very large quantities may be carcinogenic. On a toxicity scale, comfrey appears to have about the same cancer-causing potential as peanut butter, and neither should be ingested in large amounts.

Medicinal Uses; Catalysts and Combinations

The wound-healing and anti-inflammatory properties have gained comfrey wide respect as a valuable agent in promoting tissue regeneration. It is astringent in nature, which makes it very useful for bleeding in the stomach, lungs, or kidneys. It is also useful in treating hemorrhoids and uterine hemorrhaging. Comfrey is excellent for torn ligaments, bruises, and varicose veins when applied as a poultice. It makes a good gargle for throat inflammations. It has been used to treat bronchitis, asthma, sinusitis, and insect bites. As a demulcent, combine with marshmallow. It is also good combined with burdock.

Dosage and Administration
Simmer 2 teaspoons of the chopped root in 1½ cups of water. Drink once or twice a day. Or take ½ teaspoon of the tincture. Use more if treating bleeding. If using leaves, pour 1 pint of boiling water over ½ ounce of dried leaf; steep 10 minutes and strain.

Gathering and Useful Notes
Roots should be dug in either spring or autumn and the roots split down the middle. Leaves should be dried slowly. The mature leaf is safer to use as a tea, since the present controversy about use of comfrey internally has focused on the root and very young leaves. It is perfectly safe as a poultice, which is made by simmering fresh root until it forms a thick mash, and then spreading it on a linen cloth and applying it to the wound.

History and Lore
Comfrey was called "knitbone" because of the increased speed at which broken bones and wounds healed when applied externally. When comfrey paste cools it gets hard, like plaster, and therefore it was used as the earliest primitive casts. It was a favorite healing plant of the Cherokee. The Greeks believed the juice was magic because it made torn flesh mend once again. Comfrey was considered useful in attracting money, and the root was worn to protect one when traveling. It was long believed that, added to bath water, it acted as a skin rejuvenator.

Correspondences
  Planet: Saturn
  Element: Earth
  Gender: Female
  Sign: Capricorn

Cramp Bark

High cranberry, black haw

The herb is a perennial bush that grows in the U.S. in woods and foothills. It has a straight stem, four to twelve feet high, and thin bark, slightly gray in color, and splintered scales. The leaves are three-lobed and wedged; the flowers are large and white, tinged with green or red. The fruit looks like cranberries.

Part used: Dried bark

Therapeutic Profile

Antispasmodic
Analgesic
Nervine
Astringent
Emmenagogue

Recent Research

Animal studies indicate that cramp bark reduces blood pressure and strengthens heart muscle contraction. Studies also demonstrate that, after stimulation of the uterus with estrogen injections, extracts of the herb significantly inhibit the action, thus serving as a smooth muscle relaxant.

Medicinal Uses; Catalysts and Combinations

Cramp bark is highly antispasmodic and it is considered an excellent relaxing herb for menstrual cramps and nervous conditions of a hormonal nature. It is a valuable ally for a pre-menopausal woman who is flooding or having extremely heavy periods. It provides a rich supply of hormonal precursors. It protects a woman during pregnancy from miscarriage and has been used to treat asthma and a variety of nervous disorders. It is combined with wild yam, dong quai, or false unicorn root for hormonal balance, and with valerian for a sedative effect.

Dosage and Administration
Put 2 teaspoons of the bark in 1½ cups water; bring to a boil and simmer 10 minutes. Drink 2–4 times a day. Use 10–20 drops of the tincture as needed, or take up to 4–8 capsules a day for cramps.

Gathering and Useful Notes
The bark is stripped in early summer before the profuse flowers begin to bloom in June. Cut into small pieces and dry. A formula given by Dr. Christopher can be made with cramp bark, yam, skullcap, vervain, and cloves for hormone balance. Simmer all ingredients slowly for 30 minutes and add 4 ounces of glycerin; take 1–2 teaspoons in warm water.

History and Lore
Cramp bark, often called black haw, was widely used by North American Indians as a uterine tonic, and early American physicians became very proficient in recommending it to women for a variety of female complaints. In Canada and the U.S. in the nineteenth century, it was frequently used to halt a threatened abortion. Although it is often admired for its deep red clusters of berries, they are poisonous. It was often planted throughout Britain to denote property borders.

Correspondences
    Planet: Moon
    Element: Water
    Gender: Female
    Sign: Cancer

Damiana
Aphrodisiaca

Damiana is a small shrub that is indigenous to Mexico and parts of the western U.S. It has thin, branching stems with pointed, serrated leaves, and small, pale white flowers that perch on the edges of the leaf at the place where it meets the stem.

Parts used: Leaves and stems

Therapeutic Profile
Antidepressant
Diuretic
Laxative
Antiseptic
Tonic
Aperient

Recent Research
Clinical studies have found the herb to be beneficial for nervous tension and mental exhaustion. However, research has not upheld its purported effects as an aphrodisiac.

Medicinal Uses; Catalysts and Combinations
Damiana is principally a nervous system stimulant, which is why it may be thought of as a sexual stimulant. It does have a tonic effect on the hormonal system. It is used as a mild antidepressant. The hormonal effects are balancing for both men and women. It is useful in relieving constipation and bloating, and it is good for treating mental and physical fatigue. It is probably something of a myth that it treats frigidity, but it has been found useful for menopause or midlife lethargy. It combines well with dong quai, ginseng, saw palmetto, and gotu kola.

Dosage and Administration

Crush 1 teaspoon of the dried leaf and pour 1 cup boiling water over it; steep 10 minutes. Drink 2–3 times a day, or take 10–30 drops of the tincture. Capsules may be taken 1–3 times a day.

Gathering and Useful Notes

Gather the whole plant right when it begins to flower. Dry the leaves and stems slowly. Damiana tea may be drunk freely as an aphrodisiac if desired, for unlike numerous other reputed aphrodisiacs, it has been demonstrated to be safe. The leaves may be used to flavor liqueurs.

History and Lore

Damiana has a history of being an aphrodisiac since the 1800s, when it was introduced into American medicine and sold as an expensive tincture. The myths surrounding it were based, in part, on stories of Mexican fathers who had sired children at very advanced ages. It is thought by some to increase psychic ability and clairvoyance. According to folklore, it should be stored with a piece of quartz. When used in meditation, it is thought to generate mental visual imagery. It is a legendary brain tonic.

Correspondences

    Planet: Pluto
    Element: Water
    Gender: Female
    Sign: Scorpio

Dandelion

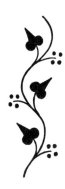

Crankwort, lion's tooth, wild endive

Dandelion is a wild perennial that grows most everywhere. It has oblong, irregular, saw-toothed leaves, and milky white juice at the stem. Its yellow flowers close at sunset. It has a globular puffball that is easily dissipated.

Parts used: Root, leaves

Therapeutic Profile
Hepatic
Cholagogue
Diuretic
Aperient
Tonic
Nutritive

Recent Research
In animal studies dandelion stimulates the flow of bile and in clinical trials it improves liver congestion and gall stones. Preliminary studies are exploring the possibility of its use as an insulin substitute.

Medicinal Uses; Catalysts and Combinations
Dandelion is an extremely rich nutrient and is considered one of the best blood builders. One cup contains 7,000 units of vitamin A. It has been used to clear the gallbladder and treat jaundice. The herb is a strong diuretic and even though diuretics tend to rob the body of potassium, dandelion is one of the strongest sources for this mineral. It is a very mild laxative and, taken prior to menstruation, can help prevent bloating. Complementary agents include milk thistle or burdock for liver and gallbladder, and yarrow for water retention.

Dosage and Administration
Pour 1 pint of boiling water over 1 ounce dried leaf; steep 10–15 minutes. Drink as often as you wish. To make a decoction of the root, put 2–3 teaspoons of chopped root in 1–2 cups water, bring to boil, and simmer 15 minutes. Drink hot. Or take 1 teaspoon of the tincture several times a day.

Gathering and Useful Notes
Collect leaves during the flowering and collect roots in the fall. They are best when they are most bitter. The roots should be split open and dried. When in season, the leaves are good in salads.

History and Lore
Dandelion has been widely regarded in both East and West for centuries. It was used by ancient Chinese Ayurvedic healers. The common name "lion's tooth" comes from the French *dent de lion* and is based on the resemblance of the jagged leaves. It is attributed to the sun because its golden-colored flower closes at night and opens only with the return of the sun. In ancient times, it was thought that all plants with yellow flowers stimulated yellow bile for the liver. In this case, it is indeed true. In folklore, it was believed to increase one's psychic abilities. The Irish call it heart-fever grass and it is drunk to overcome despondency.

Correspondences
Planet: Sun
Element: Fire
Gender: Male
Sign: Leo

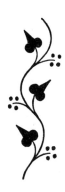

Dong Quai

Tang kwei, angelica root

Both kinds of angelica, found in the East and the West, have a round, grooved stem, branched near the top, growing three to seven feet high. The leaves grow from sheaths that surround the stem. The lower leaves are bi- or tri-ternately divided or incised; the upper are often three cleft or single. Roots are brown or gray.

Part used: Root

Therapeutic Profile

Emmenagogue
Stimulant
Tonic
Alternative
Analgesic
Antispasmodic

Recent Research

Isolated components of the herb have been shown to have a stimulating effect on the uterus; the herb is estrogenic in nature. Studies also indicate that it improves circulation. It is being investigated for its role in lowering blood pressure.

Medicinal Uses; Catalysts and Combinations

Dong quai is a very popular herbal remedy for women and is sometimes called "the female ginseng." It is used to correct painful or irregular menstruation and it facilitates hormonal balance for women in menopause. Women find it particularly helpful for hot flashes and insomnia. It helps prevent spasms, relaxes the blood vessels, purifies the blood, and is a circulatory stimulant. Regular use helps prevent anemia and can normalize blood pressure. Complementary agents include black cohosh, cramp bark, sarsaparilla, damiana, and licorice for PMS and menopause.

Dosage and Administration

The herb is most easily taken in tincture or capsules. Take 1 teaspoon of the tincture 2–3 times a day, or 1–2 capsules twice a day. There are some excellent Chinese commercial tonics available that contain dong quai.

Gathering and Useful Notes

Roots should be gathered in the spring. Dong quai is from the species of angelica known as *Angelica sinensis*. The Western herb, *Angelica archangelica*, can sometimes be substituted, as it also reduces cramping and is a warming agent. Do not use during pregnancy. Do not use in case of fibroids or excess bleeding. Dong quai will increase menstrual flow, and may cause diarrhea in some people.

History and Lore

The herb is sometimes referred to as angelica root. In the West it is associated with the archangel of healing, who in the Middle Ages appeared in a dream to a monk and revealed it as an herb that would cure many diseases and be one of the best protective measures against spirits of pestilence. It was sprinkled in all the corners of the home to protect from infection, poisons, and mad dogs. *Angelica sinensis* (dong quai) has been used for thousands of years in China, where it is second in popularity only to ginseng. It is said to have yin qualities, however, as opposed to the yang principles of ginseng.

Correspondences

Planet: Venus
Element: Water
Gender: Female
Sign: Pisces

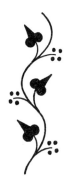

Echinacea

Purple coneflower, sampson root

The herb grows primarily in the northern U.S. on open prairies. It has a hairy, sturdy stem and linear tapering leaves, with large purple flowers that grow in ray-like petals over a raised conical disk.

Parts used: Root, flowers

Therapeutic Profile

Immunostimulant
Anti-inflammatory
Antibiotic
Alternative
Tonic

Recent Research

Laboratory research has isolated the compounds in echinacea responsible for fighting infections and stimulating the thymus gland. It stimulates the body's production of interferon, which may help the body fight cancer and herpes, as well as all manner of viruses.

Medicinal Uses; Catalysts and Combinations

Traditionally, echinacea has been used as a blood purifier, particularly for skin conditions and for fever. It can be used for boils, burns, canker sores, eczema, and acne. It is an excellent overall tonic with slightly warming qualities. Taken during the early part of flu season, it strengthens the body from invasion by germs. Echinacea also helps release toxins and is a useful lymph cleanse. It normalizes the white blood cell count and destroys bacteria and worms. It is recommended for viral and yeast infections, and for arthritic pains. It appears to have a cortisone-like action that makes it useful as an anti-inflammatory. Echinacea is good combined with cayenne, cat's claw, and goldenseal for immune enhancement.

Dosage and Administration

Put 1–2 teaspoons of the chopped root in 1½ cups of water, bring to a boil, and simmer 15 minutes. Take 1 tablespoon 3–6 times a day or 15–30 drops of the tincture every few hours, or 2–4 capsules several times a day when fighting infections.

Gathering and Useful Notes

Both *Echinacea angustifolia* and *Echinacea purpurea* should be dug up the second year or later. The roots should be unearthed in the fall and, if possible, a fresh extract squeezed as soon as possible. If the root stock is dried, it should not be used once it has lost its odor. Leaves can be gathered any time. They dry quickly and should be immediately stored. It is best used intermittently and works well if taken at the onset of an infection. The herb may produce a tingling sensation on the tongue.

History and Lore

Echinacea has enjoyed great popularity as a miracle herb and in the nineteenth century was patented as a "snake oil." One story told of a peddler who actually traveled with a live rattlesnake to a pharmaceutical institute where he let the snake bite him; he then cured himself with echinacea to demonstrate its worth. It is one of the most widely used herbs in Europe and is imported in great quantities. In folklore, the root was often worn as a strengthening agent. The American Indians used it as an offering to spirits and, in a more practical vein, to cure snakebites. (Perhaps there was more to the snake oil legends than just a huckster's wild yarn.) In Germany, extensive research the past two decades has demonstrated echinacea's having a host of infection-fighting properties.

Correspondences
  Planet: Mercury
  Element: Air
  Gender: Male
  Sign: Gemini

English Walnut

Black walnut, oil nut, walnut

The tree is large and spreading, sixty to eighty feet high, with dark, glossy leaves and dark bark with fibers running through it. It has a dark-colored nut, about one and a half inches long, and an oily kernel, pleasantly aromatic.

Parts used: Hulls, leaves, bark

Therapeutic Profile

Astringent

Tonic

Laxative

Recent Research

Several constituents have been isolated in the herb that appear to have anticancer properties. Recent research also suggests that it has antiseptic and antifungal activity.

Medicinal Uses; Catalysts and Combinations

English walnut has been used in the treatment of parasitic infections, skin diseases, and worms. It is useful for athlete's foot, yeast infections, cold sores, and gum diseases. Recently it has shown promise in treating candida and herpes. It can be used to check milk production. The bark is an excellent astringent for canker sores and boils. It also counteracts poison oak toxins and is a bug repellent. English walnut is a general tonic for blood cleansing, and useful for constipation. It can be combined with garlic and rose hips as an antioxidant and with *Cascara sagrada* as a laxative.

Dosage and Administration

Make a tea of the leaves and bark by pouring 1 cup of boiling water over 2 teaspoons of the herb; steep 15 minutes. Take 1 cup a day. As a tincture, take 5–10 drops 2 or 3 times daily.

Gathering and Useful Notes

The leaf tea is a good tonic if taken separately from the bark. A syrup can be made from the bark alone by boiling 1 pound bark in water and evaporating the solution down to 1 pint. Add sugar or honey till it reaches desired sweetness. Boil until it reaches a thick consistency. Do not take if nursing.

History and Lore

English walnut was believed to strengthen the heart if carried or worn. It was also thought to attract lightening. It has enjoyed the reputation of expelling worms by both the Asians and American Indians. It was once a common dye for the hair, and was given to check dandruff. Walnut trees were thought to be a favorite haunt of witches, who danced around them after midnight. It was considered good luck to receive a bag of walnuts from a friend. It was also regarded as a useful insect repellent.

Correspondences

Planet: Sun
Element: Fire
Gender: Male
Sign: Leo

Eyebright

Red eyebright, euphrasy

Eyebright is a small annual common to meadows and pastures. It has a square stem around twelve inches high with opposite, ovate leaves that are very stiff. The flowers are two-lipped and come in many colors. The roots are twisted and dark brown.

Parts used: All of the herb above ground

Therapeutic Profile

Astringent
Anti-inflammatory
Decongestant
Tonic
Expectorant

Recent Research

There is little research that has been done with this herb, although many positive clinical cases are reported by doctors in treating sore, inflamed eyes or conjunctivitis. Its mode of action is unknown.

Medicinal Uses; Catalysts and Combinations

Eyebright has long been used to treat eye ailments, especially red, inflamed eyes and pink eye (conjunctivitis). It is a useful remedy for problems of mucous membranes and congestive states such as nasal catarrh and sinusitis. It has been used for glaucoma and weak eyesight due to aging, as well as normal eyestrain. As a secondary use, it can be combined with bilberry and grape seed its tonic action.

Dosage and Administration

To take internally, prepare an infusion by pouring 1 cup of boiling water over 1 teaspoon of dried leaves; steep 10 minutes. Up to 3 capsules a day may be taken.

Gathering and Useful Notes

Gather while the herb is in bloom in late summer or early fall. To make an eye compress, boil the aerial parts of the herb for 10 minutes. When used as a compress for the eyes, do not use the powdered herb; use the whole plant. Leave the compress on the eyes for 15–20 minutes.

History and Lore

Eyebright has been in use for at least 2,000 years in the treatment of eye problems, and the Doctrine of Signatures shows that there is a close relationship between the name and its properties. To the English, eyebright was a symbol of fidelity. Dr. Christopher developed an eyebright formula that healed many cases of glaucoma, cataracts, and, in at least one case, blindness. One young man had been blind for ten years. Although eyebright is something of a legend, so is Dr. Christopher. Many great healers are mediums for grace to enter the world. Dr. Christopher was a devoted, prayerful man, and how much of his healing power was solely herbal has indeed sparked the interest of a number of us who are deeply indebted to the contributions of this great man.

Correspondences

    Planet: Mars
    Element: Fire
    Gender: Male
    Sign: Aries

$\mathcal{F}$alse Unicorn Root

Blazing star, drooping starwort

The plant has smooth, angular stems, one to two feet high, and rosettes of leaves that are four to eight inches long and broad-shaped. The flowers are white, tinged with green, very small and prolific, clustered in plumes. The roots are gray-brown, one-half to one inch long, and nearly cylindrical.

Part used: Root

Therapeutic Profile
Reproductive Tonic
Diuretic
Emmenagogue
Emetic

Recent Research
The principal constituent in false unicorn root is a steroidal saponin, which appears to have a normalizing function on the ovaries.

Medicinal Uses; Catalysts and Combinations
The herb has traditionally been used as a uterine tonic, but it is strengthening to the reproductive organs in both women and men. It is good for treating mucous membranes, and has been used for loss of appetite, unless too much is taken, whereupon it has the opposite effect. It is particularly helpful in cases of irregular menstruation and for ovarian pains. It is also frequently used for infertility. Diuretic in one of its actions, it is good for urinary tract infections, especially when combined with juniper and yarrow. For estrogen-like effects, use with black cohosh and licorice.

Dosage and Administration

Put 1–2 teaspoons of the dried root in 1–2 cups of water, bring to a boil, and simmer for 10–15 minutes. Drink 2–3 times a day. Or take 10–20 drops of tincture 3 times daily, or 2 capsules 3 times daily.

Gathering and Useful Notes

False unicorn root (*Helonias opulus*) is not to be confused with *Helonias bullata,* now considered an endangered species. It also should not be confused with true unicorn root, although it resembles it. Dr. Christopher considered false unicorn root a more superior herb for use as a female tonic. For treating irregular menstrual cycles, best results are obtained after at least a three-month period of use.

History and Lore

Folklore tells us that the root was used as a protection against evil spirits and was carried during travels. The sign of the cross was made with it just outside doorways. The herb was introduced by the North American tribes to early settlers, who used it as a female tonic with squaw root (black cohosh). They called it "devil's bit;" the name came from a myth that a demon tried to take a bite of the root but was frightened off by the healing spirit within. False unicorn root was used by Dr. Christopher several times to aid in a successful pregnancy where there had been previous miscarriages.

Correspondences

Planet: Venus
Element: Earth
Gender: Female
Sign: Taurus

*F*enugreek
Greek hay

Fenugreek is an annual plant with a long root, native to the Mediterranean. There are very few branches and numerous trifoliate leaves, slightly hairy. It has yellow or white flowers, often tinged with blue, and a many-seeded compressed legume.

Part used: Seeds

Therapeutic Profile
Bitter
Expectorant
Demulcent
Galactagogue

Recent Research
Clinical studies show that fenugreek reduces cholesterol and lowers blood sugar. French scientists found that it stimulates pancreatic secretion. One study suggests it may be an effective spermicidal agent.

Medicinal Uses; Catalysts and Combinations
Fenugreek is an ancient medicinal for treating bronchitis, coughs, and lung infections. It is a soothing mucilaginous herb for alleviating mucus congestion in both the lungs and the gastrointestinal tract. It helps control cellulite formation and is added to drinks to increase fiber in the diet. It may help regulate insulin production and is good for digestion. Fenugreek makes an excellent gargle for sore throats. It is also estrogenic in nature and may be used as part of a menopausal diet. Complementary agents include dandelion, myrrh, and red clover.

Dosage and Administration
Use 2 teaspoons of the seed per cup of cold water, and let stand several hours. Heat and boil 1–2 minutes. Take 2–3 cups per day. As a tincture, take 10–20 drops 3 times a day.

Gathering and Useful Notes
Fenugreek flowers about three to four weeks after the young annuals are planted, and in another three weeks it goes to seed. Seed pods should be harvested when fully formed. Remove the seeds and dry in the sun, then grind to make a poultice.

History and Lore
Fenugreek is one of the oldest herbal medicines, used by the ancient Egyptians, and highly esteemed by the Greeks and Romans. The latter thought of it as an aphrodisiac and also used it as a culinary agent. It was mentioned by Hippocrates. It has a reputation not only for the stimulation of milk production but also in the development of breasts. Arab women ate it to gain weight, since that culture's beauty standards were not defined by Hollywood trimness. It was often fed to sick animals, mixing it in with the hay—hence the name "Greek hay." An old folk remedy is to soak the seeds in water and apply to warts to make them disappear. A few seeds left in an open jar in the home was supposed to increase cash flow.

Correspondences
Planet: Mercury
Element: Earth
Gender: Female
Sign: Virgo

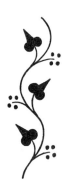

Garlic
Stinkweed

Garlic is a perennial with a compound bundle of bulbs enclosed together in a thin skin. It has a strong, straight, round stem with tubular leaf sheaths clustered at the bottom. The leaves are long, flat, and linear, and the flowers small and white.

Part used: Bulb

Therapeutic Profile
Antiseptic
Antibiotic
Antioxidant
Anti-inflammatory
Carminative
Cholagogue
Expectorant
Pectoral
Febrifuge

Recent Research
There have been more than 700 studies on garlic over the past thirty years, and at least 200 compounds isolated that have been proven beneficial for cholesterol, blood pressure, and protection against bacteria, radiation, and free radicals.

Medicinal Uses; Catalysts and Combinations
Garlic is one of the most widely used garden herbs, suited for a variety of needs. It is an excellent microbial and keeps the body free from bacteria and parasites. It is a good tonic for digestion and a useful expectorant for coughs and bronchitis. It helps regularize the liver and gallbladder. Garlic is a very important preventive herbal food as well, especially for keeping cholesterol and blood pressure in check. An extract is useful in treating intestinal worms. It is the best home

cold remedy and will help bring down fevers. Use with echinacea, cayenne, and goldenseal for treating infections.

Dosage and Administration
Juice may be pressed from the bulb and added to food or drinks. For coughs, take grated garlic with a little honey. Capsules are available and can be taken several times a day when fighting infections. A clove may be taped to an infant's foot and the benefits will find its way into the body.

Gathering and Useful Notes
Gather the bulbs when the leaves begin to brown and wither in the fall. Keep in a cool, dry place. A homemade tincture of this fine common garden herb can be made by soaking ½ pound of the peeled cloves in 1 quart of brandy for 2 weeks in a sealed container and shaking a few times a day. Then strain. The tincture will keep about a year. Take 1 teaspoon every 2–4 hours if fighting infections.

History and Lore
Garlic is a very old herb, thought to be used by the Egyptians for strength in building the pyramids. The Bible mentions that the Israelites used it. Roman soldiers ate it in the belief that it inspired courage. It was often strung on necklaces as an amulet. The mythical Odysseus used it to keep the witch Circe from turning him into a pig. In many places, it is thought to be a powerful charm against the evil eye. Garlic has the power to destroy a magnet's power of attraction, if rubbed on it (i.e., we tend to think the power of attraction is destroyed by garlic breath)! On the other hand, a garlic clove hammered into the wall of a business place was said to attract customers. It is said to be the "Russian penicillin."

Correspondences
  Planet: Mars
  Element: Fire
  Gender: Male
  Sign: Aries

Gentian
Bitter root, bitterwort

Yellow gentian grows almost five feet tall, with large, many-veined, oval-shaped leaves that terminate in a sharp point. The roots are many-branched and thin; the flowers are a bright yellow, with large plumes. Tibetan gentian has large fleshy leaves that droop like tongues.

Parts used: Root (yellow), leaves (Tibetan)

Therapeutic Profile
Bitter
Cholagogue
Hepatic
Stimulant
Anti-inflammatory

Recent Research
Gentian has been found to stimulate the flow of saliva, gastric juices, and bile. One study demonstrated that it has anti-inflammatory activity.

Medicinal Uses; Catalysts and Combinations
Gentian has principally been used as a bitter, to stimulate appetite and facilitate digestion. The flavor is very strong but, unlike many bitters, it has no astringent effects and contains no tannin. It will stimulate the secretion of bile and therefore is beneficial for gallbladder problems. It is an excellent tonic for the entire digestive tract; effective for gas, heartburn, gastritis, and healing to the pancreas. The Chinese used it for arthritic pain. It causes the stimulation of the uterus and therefore tends to promote menstruation. It is useful when combined with ginger for digestion.

Dosage and Administration
Shred ½ teaspoon into 1½ cups of water, and simmer for about 5–10 minutes. Drink before meals. Or take the tincture, 10–30 drops, as needed for digestion.

Gathering and Useful Notes
Dig the roots in the fall and cut lengthwise. Dry slowly, for to dry them too quickly will kill the bitter odor and taste that are so effective medicinally. If harvested correctly, the bitter flavor of gentian is so intense that it persists in dilutions of 1 part per 20,000. Use only in small amounts and add a flavoring agent. Cut back if it causes stomach irritation. Leaves of Tibetan gentian may be eaten raw or drunk as a tea. Wild yellow gentian, like many roots, is becoming endangered, and eco-herbalists should attempt to use the Tibetan and cultivated varieties instead.

History and Lore
The name "gentian" comes from a second-century king of Illyria, Gentius, who was credited with first discovering it. However, 1,000 years earlier, it was used by the Egyptians. In folklore, it was believed that if part of the root was in one's wallet or purse, it would protect one from pickpockets. In some places, it is chewed as a substitute for tobacco. For quite some time, it was used in brewing beer, before the discovery of hops. It is Europe's most important bitter.

Correspondences
    Planet: Mars
    Element: Water
    Gender: Male
    Sign: Scorpio

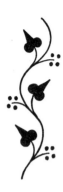

Ginger
African ginger, black ginger, Asian ginger

Ginger grows primarily in tropical areas. It has a simple leafy stem covered with sheaths of oblong pointed leaves around six to ten inches long. The root is knotty, fibrous, and pleasing to smell. It grows to a height of three to four feet and has white and yellow flowers with purple streaks.

Part used: Root

Therapeutic Profile
Diaphoretic
Antibiotic
Carminative
Stimulant
Rubefacient
Anti-inflammatory

Recent Research
Numerous studies have been conducted demonstrating ginger's effectiveness, over the more commonly used drugs, in treating nausea. It has anti-inflammatory effects and has been shown to lower blood pressure and cholesterol. Several components have been isolated that are antibiotic in nature.

Medicinal Uses; Catalysts and Combinations
Ginger is an excellent toxin cleanser, promoting cleansing through perspiration and circulation. It promotes good digestion and wards off infections. It is useful in treating colds, sore throats, and fevers, as well as colic, gas, and diarrhea. It is good for motion sickness or morning sickness. Recent studies that demonstrate its efficacy as a natural anti-inflammatory tend to verify why it has been used for centuries to treat joint problems. Ginger is often eaten after meals

and protects against indigestion and gastritis. It has been used as an effective headache reliever. Use with cayenne for cleansing and colds.

Dosage and Administration

Pour 1 cup of boiling water over 1 teaspoon of fresh root; steep 5 minutes. Drink as often as desired, or mix ½ teaspoon of the powdered root with 1 teaspoon honey and add hot water. In tincture form, take 10–15 drops several times a day, or take 3–4 capsules a day.

Gathering and Useful Notes

Gather roots after the leaves have withered. Wash well and dry in the sun. A decoction can be made by chopping the root in small pieces and simmering 2 teaspoons per cup for 10 minutes. The rootstock may be chewed as it is, or candied and eaten after meals. It is very safe, even for children.

History and Lore

Ginger has a 3,000-year-old history in China, prescribed for flu, hangover, respiratory illness, and kidney problems. The West only recently discovered that it is an effective aid for nausea. Many ancient cultures used it to preserve food. In India it was believed that eating ginger made one smell sweet, and therefore a devotee was more appealing to the gods. The Greeks first used it for gingerbread. In the Caribbean it is thought to increase fertility. Sometimes it was chewed and spat out to expel sickness.

Correspondences
  Planet: Mars
  Element: Fire
  Gender: Male
  Sign: Aries

Ginkgo

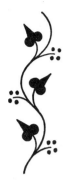

Maidenhair tree, golden fossil tree

Ginkgo is a large tree, growing to eighty feet, and very large at the base. The small stems growing off the main branches divide and terminate in delicate fan-shaped leaves, with alternate numerous berry-shaped nuts, very small, also growing close to the main branches.

Parts used: Leaves, seeds

Therapeutic Profile

Stimulant

Cardiotonic

Bitter

Antioxidant

Astringent

Alternative

Expectorant

Recent Research

The ginkgo leaf contains flavonoid, its valuable antioxidant property. The extract has a strong affinity for the adrenals and the central nervous system, and studies show it improves circulation and flow of blood to the brain. Its anti-aggregatory effect on platelets may offer protection against strokes.

Medicinal Uses; Catalysts and Combinations

Although the nut has primarily been used in Chinese medicine, the recent interest in the herb in the West has concentrated on an extract of the leaves. Traditionally, the nut was used for asthma, bronchitis, and pulmonary conditions. The leaf is effective for peripheral blood circulation and increased circulatory oxygenation to the brain cells. It is now used to treat attention deficit disorders, Alzheimer's, blood clots, memory loss, stroke, tinnitus, and vascular disease. It is useful in reducing anxiety, alleviating headache, and improving vision in some people. Ginkgo is one of the most excellent herbal preventives against senility. Complementary agents include ginseng and gotu kola.

Dosage and Administration
Commercial preparations are commonly available. In tincture form, take ½ to 1 teaspoon 3 times a day, or 2–3 capsules a day.

Gathering and Useful Notes
Hang the leaves upside down in the shade to dry, then store immediately. Do not use if you have blood-clotting disorders. Do not use with children except for treating asthma. Large doses may cause diarrhea or irritability. Ginkgo needs to be used regularly for several months to be effective for memory.

History and Lore
Ginkgo is the world's oldest living tree species, demonstrating again a relationship to the Doctrine of Signatures, since it is known as a longevity herb. It was nearly destroyed in the Ice Age, but survived in China. The Chinese and Japanese roasted the seeds and used it as a prevention for drunkenness. In India, it was thought of as the magical "soma" elixir. It was not introduced into Europe until the eighteenth century, and did not grow in popularity until this century. Its cultivation has spread throughout the world, but in the East it is still considered a sacred tree. It lives 2,000 years or more. Ginkgo is one of the most widely prescribed herbal medicines in Europe, with sales skyrocketing over $500 million a year.

Correspondences
    Planet: Saturn
    Element: Air
    Gender: Male
    Sign: Capricorn

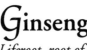

Ginseng
Liferoot, root of immortality

Siberian ginseng (eleuthero) is a spring shrub native in woodland areas of Siberia and Korea. American ginseng (Panax) is a herbaceous perennial that grows easily in the forests of North America. It has thin stems with five to six veined leaves each. Ginseng roots generally are multi-branched and fleshy. They have numerous limbs attached to the main root. The tiny flowers cluster near the main stem.

Part used: Root

Therapeutic Profile
Adaptogen
Immunostimulant
Antioxidant
Demulcent
Stimulant
Cardiotonic
Anti-inflammatory

Recent Research
Studies on Siberian ginseng show a reduction in general fatigue in up to 90 percent of patients studied or significant reduction in blood pressure in almost as many cases, demonstrating that it is superior to Asian ginseng. Studies on the latter do demonstrate some reduction in cholesterol and blood sugar levels as well.

Medicinal Uses; Catalysts and Combinations
In China, ginseng is considered the king of all tonics, providing stimulation to the whole body and offering protection against fatigue and disease in general. It is good for inflammation, fever, hormonal imbalances, and reducing blood pressure and anemia. It has been used to treat diabetes. A daily tea is said to have rejuvenating powers; certainly it is a stimulant for the central nervous system and the

endocrine glands. Its demulcent effects make it soothing for mucous membranes. It also helps to regulate blood sugar. New studies show it may be effective for heart protection and cancer. Use with gotu kola.

Dosage and Administration
Use about ½ to 1 teaspoon in 1½ cups of water, bring to a boil, and simmer 10 minutes. Drink 2 cups per day. Many commercial capsules are available; follow the directions on the bottle.

Gathering and Useful Notes
Roots take at least six years to mature and should not be harvested early. They should be unearthed carefully, so the root limbs do not break off, and dried for at least a month. Use the root as a powder. The bulk of studies show that Siberian ginseng, although not really a part of the ginseng family, is superior as an immune stimulant. Use with caution if pregnant.

History and Lore
The name "man root" comes from the belief that the roots, with their attached limbs, resemble a human being. The Chinese named it "root of immortality" because of its kinship with the gods. As its popularity spread, the once-plentiful supply became almost decimated. It is now cultivated very carefully and seeds cost almost $100 a pound. In eighteenth-century American folklore, it was thought that ginseng scared spirits away. The American Indians learned about its valuable medicinal properties from the Jesuits, who valued it as an export, along with rare furs. The Latin name *panax* means "panacea." The Panax or Asian variety is considered to be male, or yang. If it comes into contact with metal, its strength is decreased. Siberian ginseng is used by Soviet cosmonauts for alertness in space.

Correspondences
  Planet: Mars
  Element: Fire
  Gender: Male
  Sign: Aries

Goldenseal
Indian plant, yellowroot

Goldenseal is a small perennial with a hairy stem that grows about a foot high, with two slightly hairy five-lobed serrated leaves. The single flower is white or rose-colored and sits at the top of the stem. The fruit is two-seeded and resembles a raspberry. The yellow root is only two inches long, with many small rootlets.

Parts used: Root, leaves

Therapeutic Profile
Tonic
Alternative
Pectoral
Decongestant
Hepatic
Bitter
Antibiotic
Vulnerary
Immunostimulant

Recent Research
Both antiviral and antibacterial components have been documented with goldenseal. In animal studies it has lowered blood pressure. One of its primary constituents, berberine, acts as an anti-inflammatory. In one epidemic of cholera in India it was more effective than antibiotics.

Medicinal Uses; Catalysts and Combinations
Goldenseal's principal reputation has been as a tonic for gastric and genito-urinary disorders. It has been used as a tea rinse to relieve bleeding gums and canker sores and as a gargle for sore throats. The herb has a powerful immune stimulant activity and it is often used in place of antibiotics. It is effective in the treatment of any mucous membranes, and is especially good for upper respiratory congestion. Goldenseal can

be used as an eyewash and has wound-healing properties when applied externally. It stimulates uterine contractions at the onset of labor. Use with echinacea and garlic in warding off colds and infections, and with chamomile and meadowsweet for stomach problems.

Dosage and Administration
Simmer 1 teaspoon of the ground or chopped root, or root-leaf combination, in 1½ cups of water 10–15 minutes; let stand until cold. Take 2 teaspoons several times a day. Or take 5–30 drops of the extract. Up to 6 powdered capsules may be taken a day.

Gathering and Useful Notes
Roots should be unearthed and sliced lengthwise when the plant is five to seven years old, after seeds have ripened. Leaves can be harvested in late summer. Keep the root in a dry place and grind when necessary. Store infusion in a closed container. For an eyewash, add 1 teaspoon rootstock and 1 teaspoon of boric acid to 1 pint of boiling water; pour off the liquid. Add 1 teaspoon to ½ cup of water. Do not take continuously. Do not take if pregnant. Goldenseal habitats are shrinking, and cultivation of the plant is encouraged.

History and Lore
Goldenseal was widely used by Indians of the Northeast for skin diseases. The Cherokee used it for ulcers, face paint, and arrow wounds. The early settlers adopted it in the nineteenth century and it was a popular wound treatment during the Civil War. It was popularized as a medical wonder tonic and harvested until it nearly became extinct. The generic name of the plant, Hydrastis, is derived from two Greek meanings that signify "water" and "accomplishment," no doubt because of its effect on the mucous membranes. Goldenseal was a very popular herb among the common people and was often called "poor man's ginseng."

Correspondences
   Planet: Sun
   Element: Fire
   Gender: Male
   Sign: Leo

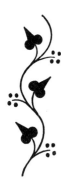

Gotu Kola
Indian pennywort, marshpenny

Grown primarily in Ceylon and Java, the herb should not be confused with the kola nut, which grows on a tree. Gotu kola has a creeping stem with fan-shaped leaves. It grows nears marshes and has small flowers close to the ground. The roots are thin and spindly.

Parts used: Root, leaves

Therapeutic Profile
Nervine
Tonic
Stimulant
Anti-inflammatory
Alternative
Antispasmodic
Vulnerary

Recent Research
Research indicates that gotu kola is as effective for fatigue as caffeine, but without the side effects. One study demonstrated that it accelerated healing of wounds and skin grafts. In a controlled study the herb was also effective in treating venous insufficiency.

Medicinal Uses; Catalysts and Combinations
Gotu kola has a wide range of activity, including anti-inflammatory and antibacterial. Although the herb does not contain caffeine, it is a blood stimulant and does have a rejuvenating effect if taken in small doses. In large doses, it may have the opposite (sedating) effect. It has been utilized primarily as a brain tonic and is often used in memory formulas. Prolonged use may help overcome depression, nervous conditions, and age-related disorders. It is an effective tonic for circulatory problems, high blood pressure, and arteriosclerosis. In the East,

it was used to treat leprosy and is still employed as a blood cleanser for skin diseases. It is beneficial for hormonal balance, particularly menopause, where it is combined with wild yam. Use with ginseng and ginkgo for brain rejuvenation.

Dosage and Administration
Use ½ teaspoon of the herb with 1½ cups of boiling water; simmer 10 minutes and drink 2–3 cups a day. It is available in numerous formulas in capsule form: Follow directions given for that particular formula.

Gathering and Useful Notes
Gotu kola is not cultivated in the United States, and when buying the imported herb it should not be labeled "kola nut," which is of a completely different family. It does not have caffeine effects, but it does cause restlessness or insomnia in some people; if so, discontinue use. Use as a compress for skin problems, such as psoriasis.

History and Lore
Gotu kola has a reputation for being a longevity herb in the East, probably because it was believed to be used by Liching Yun, who purportedly lived 256 years. The natives of Ceylon also associated it with a long life because their elephants, who seemed to live very long indeed, enjoyed munching on the leaves. They had a saying, "Two leaves a day keep old age away." In India, the plant is called "bramhi" or the "greatest of the great;" it is also considered the herb of enlightenment. Gotu kola is a popular Ayurvedic herb and is used frequently by the Philippine healers as well. It is sometimes used as an incense and burned during meditation.

Correspondences
   Planet: Saturn
   Element: Air
   Gender: Male
   Sign: Aquarius

Ground Ivy

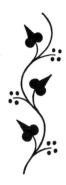

Alehoof, cat's foot, haymaids

Ground ivy is a creeping perennial common to much of Europe and the eastern U.S. It has a square stem, growing one to two feet long, with tiny hairs. The roots grow from the nodes along the stem. The leaves are also hairy, opposite, and rounded. It has bluish flowers that grow in small whorls.

Parts used: Leaves, flowers

Therapeutic Profile
Astringent
Stimulant
Expectorant
Diuretic
Carminative

Recent Research
Saponins of ivy have been demonstrated to be effective against parasites when taken internally. Studies also have been focused on the external use of the resin.

Medicinal Uses; Catalysts and Combinations
Ground ivy has been used principally for inflammation of the mucous membranes, especially for sore throat and bronchitis. It is a good appetite stimulant. It may also stimulate menstruation in some women. Applied externally, it has proven useful in treating skin ulcers and small wounds. Ground ivy is rich in vitamin C and has been used to treat scurvy. It is beneficial to both kidneys and liver. Because of its astringency, it is useful in curing diarrhea. It is a safe herb to use for children's stomachaches. Combine with horehound and goldenseal for sinus problems.

Dosage and Administration
Steep 1 teaspoon of the fresh herb in 1 cup of water. Drink ½ cup twice daily. It may be taken in juice or tincture, ½ teaspoon at a time.

Gathering and Useful Notes
Gather flowers and stems from April through June. Make a poultice of ground aerial parts mixed with yarrow for external use. The juice should be used for stomach complaints. It can be added to bathwater for relief of sciatica. Do not take in large amounts.

History and Lore
Ivy stems have long been used as a source of dyes, primarily dark yellow and brown tones. It was a religious vine in several Greek myths, and is particularly associated with Dionysus, who was the god of revelry. Ivy was made into wreaths and worn for initiations and celebrations. It was the crown for those who had been victorious in mock battles. Newlyweds wore it, and it came to represent fidelity. In folklore, it was said that to use it in divination would reveal the name of whomever carried a grudge against you.

Correspondences
   Planet: Mars
   Element: Water
   Gender: Female
   Sign: Scorpio

Hawthorn

Maybush, mayflower, thorn apple

Hawthorn is a common hedge plant with a trunk of gray, smooth wood and thorny branches. It is characterized by small shiny leaves, dark green on top and slightly blue underneath. It has white flowers with round petals and a red fleshy fruit with two or three leaves.

Parts used: Berries, flowers

Therapeutic Profile

Antispasmodic
Cardiotonic
Antioxidant
Sedative
Diuretic
Carminative

Recent Research

The therapeutic properties of hawthorn have been well researched. Its high bioflavonoid content dilates peripheral and coronary blood vessels. It has also been shown to lower cholesterol.

Medicinal Uses; Catalysts and Combinations

Hawthorn is famous as a heart and blood tonic. Used over time, it lowers blood pressure and will normalize heart action. It was also used by North American Indians for rheumatism and for digestive problems. Some herbalists advise it for insomnia. It is now most widely prescribed for angina, irregular heartbeat, cholesterol reduction, and hypertension. Use in the early stages of congestive heart failure. Combine with cayenne, ginkgo, and garlic.

Dosage and Administration
Steep 1 teaspoon of dried flowers in ½ to 1 cup of water. Or boil 1 teaspoon of dried or fresh berries in 1½ cups water for 10 minutes. Another way to make a strong decoction is to crush 1–2 teaspoons of dried berries in 1 cup cold water. Bring to a boil and let steep for 30 minutes. Drink twice a day. One to two capsules a day may be taken.

Gathering and Useful Notes
The tree blooms from April through June. Collect flowers when fully bloomed and odoriferous. The smell may not appear aromatic; its odor repels even bees. Use only as prescribed. Consult a health-care practitioner if blood pressure drops too much. Do not use if pregnant.

History and Lore
Mayflower was the common name for the tree that has been regarded with some awe in Europe for centuries. It was long believed to be a favorite plant of witches, and on occasion witches even turned themselves into hawthorns. In ancient Greece and Rome, it was also considered numinous, but there it was associated with love, marriage, and a happy family life. It was believed to be sacred in the Christian tradition, since in one legend the crown of thorns placed on Christ's head was from a hawthorn tree that grew outside the Mount of Olives. In some places, leaves of the tree were placed near babies to ward off evil. It is reputed to be the hedge that grew overnight around Sleeping Beauty.

Correspondences
Planet: Sun
Element: Fire
Gender: Female
Sign: Leo

Hops
Beer flower

Hops are hairy climbing plants that look similar to the grape vine. The mature vines are often twenty-five feet long, with angular stems and a branched rootstock. The leaves are rough and serrated, with three to five lobes. The flowers are yellow, tinged with green. The fruit is scaly and cone-shaped.

Part used: Fruit

Therapeutic Profile

Anti-inflammatory
Analgesic
Bitter
Febrifuge
Diuretic
Sedative
Tonic
Antispasmodic

Recent Research

The herb's sedative properties were discovered in the 1980s and isolated as a sedative chemical. It works by relaxing the smooth muscles and also by acting directly on the nervous system.

Medicinal Uses; Catalysts and Combinations

Hops are a calming agent and most often they are recommended for nerves and insomnia. It is an appetite stimulant and is useful in dispelling gas. Long taken as an antispasmodic, it is particularly good for spastic conditions associated with nerves. Its diuretic properties make it useful for treatment of water retention. Hops are also good for menstrual cramps and are somewhat hormone balancing, although not as much as other herbs. Other therapeutic applications include headaches, hyperactivity, fever, inflammation, and colon disorders. Use with valerian, or with skullcap and chamomile for a milder effect.

Dosage and Administration
Pour 1 cup of boiling water over 1 teaspoon of the dried herb; steep 10 minutes. Drink 1–2 cups, bedtime is best. It may be taken in tincture or capsules; follow directions on bottle.

Gathering and Useful Notes
When harvesting, care should be taken to preserve the golden powder that is the essence of the hops. It should be stored in a very dark place and thrown away when it turns reddish brown, or starts to smell like it is aging. Hops will occasionally cause rash or diarrhea. Do not use over prolonged periods of time.

History and Lore
It is believed that if hops are sewn into a pillow, they will help one to sleep. The dried flowers have been used to make beer and ale, a rather magical discovery that occurred in the 1500s. However, it made the beer more bitter than the British were used to and for a time it was banned by Henry VIII. Eventually, it became an important cash crop. It was used by the American Indians as a sedative, who introduced it to the settlers. In the early part of this century it was a popular tonic for most everything. "Take hops bitters three times a day, and you will have no doctors to pay," was the slogan associated with it. It was long believed to possess aphrodisiac properties.

Correspondences
   Planet: Mercury
   Element: Air
   Gender: Male
   Sign: Virgo

Horehound

Hoarhound, white horehound, bull's blood

Horehound has a stem covered with white, woolly hair and spreading branches. The leaves are heart-shaped, opposite, crinkly and gray-green. It has small cream-colored flowers occurring in dense whorls just above the upper leaves.

Parts used: Leaves, flowers

Therapeutic Profile

Expectorant
Bitter
Antispasmodic
Diaphoretic
Vulnerary

Recent Research

Horehound has been shown to directly affect respiration by dilating vessels, and its derivatives are used in many bronchial medications.

Medicinal Uses; Catalysts and Combinations

Horehound is a very popular cough remedy and its oil has excellent expectorant properties. It is valuable in treating bronchitis and whooping cough. It has been used to treat hayfever and allergies. The bitter action of the herb is an aid to digestion. Externally, it has been used to facilitate the healing of wounds. It helps eliminate toxins through the skin by promoting perspiration. In some cases, it will assist in the expulsion of afterbirth. It is a common ingredient in lozenges for coughs due to colds. Combine with marshmallow, hyssop, and lobelia for respiratory problems.

Dosage and Administration
Pour 1 cup of boiling water over 1 teaspoon of the dried herb, and steep 10 minutes. Drink 1–2 cups per day.

Gathering and Useful Notes
Gather leaves from June through September, just before the flowers are in full bloom. It often does not bloom until the second year. Dry in the shade. Horehound is best taken cold. Singers often find it helpful to sustain vocal chords or when hoarse. To make a syrup, use 1 pound dark sugar per 1 pint of the infusion. Do not give to children under two years of age.

History and Lore
The ancient Egyptians dedicated horehound to their god, Horus, who conquered the Egyptian personification of evil known as Seth. It was believed to offer protection from sorcery if worn as an amulet. It was used as an exorcism herb. Sometimes it was placed in sickrooms to expel illness. Horehound was one of the herbs taken at the celebration of the Passover by Jewish celebrants. Medieval Europeans believed it offered protection against curses. It was first used for colds by the Romans, and was one of the favorite herbs of the famous healer Hildegard of Bingen.

Correspondences
    Planet: Mercury
    Element: Air
    Gender: Male
    Sign: Gemini

Hyssop

Hyssop herb, Isopo

Hyssop is an evergreen shrub growing one to two feet high, with rod-like branches and opposite, smooth, dark green leaves. It has lavender or pink flowers, arranged in tufts on spikes at the top of the square stem.

Parts used: All of the herb above ground

Therapeutic Profile

Antispasmodic
Expectorant
Sedative
Hepatic
Diaphoretic
Vulnerary
Febrifuge
Antiseptic

Recent Research

There is some research that indicates hyssop inhibits herpes simplex, both genital sores and cold sores, when applied externally.

Medicinal Uses; Catalysts and Combinations

Hyssop is an effective antispasmodic for coughs and colds. It is an excellent expectorant for most pulmonary complaints, and makes a pleasant warm gargle. It tends to normalize blood pressure. The healing virtues of the plant are due to its volatile oils, which are particularly helpful for skin irritations, bruises, and burns. It is a potent sedative for anxiety states as well as hysteria. It is sometimes used for digestive difficulties, especially flatulence. The tincture has been helpful in the effort to stop smoking. Combine with horehound for coughs and colds.

Dosage and Administration
Pour 1 cup of water over 1–2 teaspoons of the dried herb. Drink once or twice a day, or take 1–2 teaspoons of the extract. Do not overuse.

Gathering and Useful Notes
Cut the tops in late summer and dry quickly in the sun. To use as a healing balm for the skin, bruise the green parts of the herb and apply the infusion as a poultice. Use in medicinal amounts only and not for extended periods of time.

History and Lore
Hyssop is an ancient biblical herb, used as an antiseptic and in purification rites: "Purge me with hyssop and I shall be white as snow" (Psalms 51:9). It was considered a healing balm for leprosy. It has long been used to treat external wounds and one reason cited is that penicillin thrives on hyssop leaves. However, it is most likely that the amount of antibiotic is negligible and the volatile oil is what is the effective agent. Hyssop is the most widely used purification herb around the world. It is known in folklore to be a great agent for purging evil. In the Middle Ages, it was strewn around homes to cover bad smells because of its strong, camphor-like odor. The Greek word *hyssop* means "holy herb."

Correspondences
Planet: Jupiter
Element: Fire
Gender: Male
Sign: Sagittarius

Irish Moss

Carragheen, pearl moss

Irish moss is one of a variety of seaweeds found principally in coastal areas of Ireland and France. The frond is a red-purple color.

Parts used: Whole herb

Therapeutic Profile

Expectorant
Demulcent
Immunostimulant
Anti-inflammatory
Pectoral
Emollient

Recent Research

Studies associate Irish moss with lowered blood pressure. Preliminary research focuses on its use as a demulcent and an immune stimulant. Promising research indicates that the seaweeds all seem to prevent absorption of radioactive substances and toxic metals.

Medicinal Uses; Catalysts and Combinations

Used principally for chronic lung problems and goiter, the role of Irish moss and many other seaweeds is expanding considerably in this century. Its mucilaginous nature is useful in soothing inflamed tissue as well as absorbing toxins from the bowel. Many alternative practitioners now advise it for clearing radioactive poisons—to which we have all been exposed—from the body, especially strontium 90. Irish moss can reduce appetite. It is useful in treating gastritis or ulcers. It is a superb source of minerals so necessary for the endocrine and immune systems, especially the thyroid. Combine with kelp, algae, purple dulse, or spirulina.

Dosage and Administration
Use 1 teaspoon of dried herb with 1 cup of hot water; drink twice a day. Take the dried powder in 3–6 gram capsules or in combinations with other seaweeds.

Gathering and Useful Notes
This seaweed is gathered primarily along the rocky coasts of Ireland, but can be found all along northwestern Europe. It is collected at low tide. Care should be taken not to gather from industrial areas where the moss may be contaminated.

History and Lore
Irish moss is a member of the seaweed family long popular among coastal people. It was used by the colonists in New England but it has only been a popular herb in European countries since the eighteenth century. Doctors began to notice that those living along the Atlantic coast did not have enlarged thyroid glands. In this century, it became a popular ingredient in antiwrinkle creams. It is a stabilizer in many dairy products. In one folklore custom, it was placed under rugs to attract wealth. In another, it was believed that to carry Irish moss would offer protection during travel.

Correspondences
Planet: Moon
Element: Water
Gender: Female
Sign: Pisces

Juniper
Geneva, gin plant

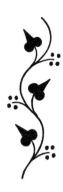

Juniper is an evergreen shrub that usually grows two to six feet high, but sometimes much higher. The bark is reddish-brown; the leaves are needle-shaped with white stripes. It has yellow and green flowers growing in whorls of three, and a berry-like, blue-black fruit.

Parts used: Berries

Therapeutic Profile
Diuretic
Carminative
Antiseptic
Stimulant
Anti-inflammatory

Recent Research
Studies with animals have demonstrated antitumor activity, and juniper also holds promise as an antiviral agent, since in cell cultures it is effective against influenza and herpes. Human studies show it alleviates arthritis.

Medicinal Uses; Catalysts and Combinations
Juniper is both a diuretic and antiseptic, and is therefore very useful in treating urinary tract infections, particularly cystitis. If there is already long-term kidney disease, it should be avoided, and marshmallow and uva ursi used instead. Juniper is good for urine retention, stones, and gravel. It has been used to soothe the stomach and eliminate flatulence and cramps. It helps to produce hydrochloric acid to aid in digestion, and it stimulates appetite. Externally, the oil is good for joint problems. Complementary agents include parsley, marshmallow, and buchu.

Dosage and Administration
Steep 1 teaspoon of the crushed berries in ½ cup of hot water for 10 minutes. Strain and drink twice a day. The dried berries may also be chewed a few at a time. Commercial oils are available. Capsules are not recommended.

Gathering and Useful Notes
Because of its volatile oil, juniper should be gathered when the berries are fully ripe but not shriveled, and then dried slowly in the shade. The oil penetrates the skin readily and should not be overused, as it may cause blisters. Do not use more than six weeks. Do not use if pregnant.

History and Lore
The American Indians used juniper root as an aid in controlling venereal disease, and strung the dried berries as beads. In Europe during the Middle Ages, the herb was regarded with awe and thought to offer protection from witches. It was planted by the front door to block their entrance. Burning the plant was seen to offer protection in averting bubonic plague. In some places a small twig of the shrub was worn as an amulet for safe travel. For over 300 years, it has been the basis of the favorite alcoholic beverage, gin, and as also used as flavoring agent for sauerkraut. Dr. Christopher's Juni-Pars became a very famous formula for urinary tract infections in the Utah hills.

Correspondences
Planet: Sun
Element: Fire
Gender: Male
Sign: Leo

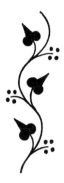

Kava-kava

Ava root, intoxicating pepper

Kava-kava is a root common to the South Pacific. It is a perennial shrub that normally grows about eight feet, with heart-shaped leaves and a woody, lined rootstock with numerous small nobs.

Part used: Root

Therapeutic Profile

Antiseptic
Antispasmodic
Sedative
Bitter
Diuretic

Recent Research

Kava has anticonvulsant and tranquilizing activity in experiments with animals. The major focus on the herb currently is for the treatment of epilepsy. Psychoactive components have also been isolated.

Medicinal Uses; Catalysts and Combinations

The root has been used where it locally grows for centuries as an analgesic sedative for the relief of pain, anxiety, or insomnia. It may be applied to wounds or taken internally. In some places it is drunk by the natives in place of alcohol and will eventually induce a stupor, if enough is consumed. It is also a diuretic and will promote cleansing through the kidneys. Kava has been used as a vaginal douche and in the treatment of venereal diseases, probably because of its antiseptic properties. The herb exerts a relaxing effect on the central nervous system. Users report greater mental clarity and improved memory. It may be combined with hops or valerian.

Dosage and Administration

Combine 4 tablespoons of the crushed root in 1 pint of water, and simmer 10 minutes. Or take 10–30 drops of the tincture. Do not overuse.

Gathering and Useful Notes

The root is dug and carefully scraped and pounded before brewing. It will initially make the mouth numb. Excessive consumption can lead to dizziness, skin rash, or liver damage. It is an effective alternative to anti-anxiety medication, however, such as Xanax and Valium, when properly used.

History and Lore

Kava is an herb surrounded by much mystique and has been used ritually by the Polynesian and Hawaiian islanders for many centuries. They valued it both as a medicine and as a ceremonial drink. Today, the rituals involving kava are open to both men and women, but its use was once reserved for men only. The women used to prepare it, however, which involved a magical method of mastication. It was believed to offer protection against demons and to entice psychic powers. It will induce visions if enough is drunk. Captain Cook gave it the name "intoxicating pepper." It is popular among European herbalists to treat anxiety.

Correspondences

Planet: Saturn
Element: Air
Gender: Female
Sign: Aquarius

Lavender

Garden lavender, elf leaf

Lavender is a very aromatic herb that grows in clumps about one to two feet high. It has thin, gray-green stems with opposite, downy leaves and lilac tubular flowers growing in whorls up the stem.

Parts used: Flowers, leaves

Therapeutic Profile

Antispasmodic
Carminative
Aromatic
Antiseptic
Anti-emetic
Nervine

Recent Research

Lavender has several components in its oil that have demonstrated antiseptic and antispasmodic properties.

Medicinal Uses; Catalysts and Combinations

Lavender is an aromatic carminative, used to relax the stomach muscles and for various digestive problems. The distilled oil is also good for nervousness, headaches, fainting, and dizziness. A leaf infusion is useful against bacteria in the intestines and it is an antiseptic when used on the skin as well. Lavender has been used to treat depression, especially in conjunction with other herbs. The oil is effective in treating the aches and pains of sore joints when rubbed into the skin. Combine with skullcap and chamomile as a tea.

Dosage and Administration

Steep 1 teaspoon of the dried leaves in 1 cup hot water. Drink once or twice a day. Commercial oil is available for external use.

Gathering and Useful Notes

Gather leaves and small buds from June through September, just before flowering. Oil rubbed into the temples is good for headache relief. It is also relaxing to add oil to bath water, or to wear it for its aromatic effects.

History and Lore

The name "lavender" comes from the Latin *lavare*, which means "to wash," perhaps because it was frequently used as a wash for skin troubles. In medieval Europe it was burned on Midsummer's Eve to enable one to invoke the spirits. Lavender is reputed to be one of the herbs used by Solomon, who had it crushed and mixed in the spring of holy water that was in his temple. It was also used in baths by the Romans. Dried buds have been collected wherever it grows and used in sachets; it is very aromatic for humans but repels insects. An old folklore legend tells us that if lavender was sprinkled over the head it would preserve one's chastity. It will also protect one from snakes.

Correspondences
Planet: Mercury
Element: Air
Gender: Male
Sign: Gemini

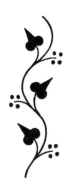

Licorice

Sweet wood, sweetroot

Licorice is a perennial plant that grows wild in many places. It has an alternate stem with ovate dark green leaves that grow in pairs. The root is brown and woody and yellow on the inside. Flowers are purple or yellow.

Part used: Root

Therapeutic Profile

Demulcent

Expectorant

Antioxidant

Immunostimulant

Anti-inflammatory

Antispasmodic

Pectoral

Nutritive

Recent Research

There has been an abundance of studies on licorice. It has estrogenic properties and it stimulates cortisone and the production of interferon. The glycyrrhizin component is famous for healing ulcers.

Medicinal Uses; Catalysts and Combinations

Licorice is famous for treating peptic ulcers, gastritis, and stomach colic. It is an excellent strengthener of the adrenals, and has been used to treat Addison's disease. Dr. Christopher used it in his famous formula for rebuilding adrenals called Adrenetone. It is very soothing to the mucous membranes and useful for all respiratory infections. It facilitates estrogen production and is frequently used in place of artificial hormones in menopause. It makes a sweet cough syrup and a medicinal candy. It has powerful anti-inflammatory properties and is good for arthritis. Sprinkling powdered root on herpes and cold sores has been found effective. Use with black cohosh and dong quai for menopause, and slippery elm for coughs.

Dosage and Administration
Use 1 teaspoon of the chopped root to 1½ cups of water, bring to boil, and simmer 10 minutes. Sip slowly. Drink twice a day. Commercial capsules come with glycyrrhizin and deglycyrrhizinated.

Gathering and Useful Notes
The plant needs to be at least four years old to harvest. Normally it is peeled, as the bark is very bitter. There are contraindications with the glycyrrhizin for some people. If it causes high blood pressure or edema, use the deglycyrrhizinated variety. Do not use if pregnant or nursing.

History and Lore
Licorice is a very popular Chinese medicine, where it was associated with longevity. It was also well-known to the Native American Indians. Among the Greeks, it was used as a thirst quencher. It makes a refreshing drink when used in flavored water. The word "licorice" is from the Greek roots *glykys*, meaning "sweet," and *rhiza*, meaning "root." The glycyrrhizic acid in licorice is fifty times sweeter than sugar. The Egyptians believed it was a sacred herb and it was stored with King Tut in his tomb as an aid on his journey to the next life. Licorice candy is sometimes used by smokers who want to stop. In folklore, it is believed that eating it will make one passionate. It is worn as an amulet for love and fidelity.

Correspondences
  Planet: Venus
  Element: Water
  Gender: Female
  Sign: Pisces

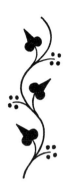

Lobelia

Gagroot, Indian tobacco

Lobelia is common to North American pastures and fields. It has a straight hairy stem, one to three feet high, with a milky sap. The leaves are thin, alternate, and slightly hairy. Lobelia has beautiful two-lipped tiny flowers, blue or white.

Parts used: Whole herb

Therapeutic Profile

Antispasmodic
Emetic
Analgesic
Expectorant
Nervine
Febrifuge
Emmenagogue

Recent Research

Lobelia will stimulate the adrenals to release corticosteroids. Studies also show that the extracts relax the smooth muscles. Clinical tests demonstrate it is an effective smoking deterrent.

Medicinal Uses; Catalysts and Combinations

Lobelia has the reputation of being a deadly plant; however, it is not poisonous if taken properly. It has a powerful relaxing effect that is nonaddictive. It has been used to treat bronchial asthma, and is an excellent expectorant. The lobelia salts make nicotine taste repulsive to the smoker and is therefore a deterrent for those who want to quit. It has been used in the treatment of epilepsy, diphtheria, and liver problems. As an antispasmodic tincture it is good for tremors, cramps, and lockjaw. It will stimulate menstrual flow and cause vomiting if taken in large amounts. Use with licorice and ginger.

Dosage and Administration

Pour 1 cup of boiling water over ¼ teaspoon of the dried herb; steep 10 minutes. Drink 1–2 times a day. Or take 5–10 drops of the tincture. In powdered form, it is best combined with other herbs.

Gathering and Useful Notes

The entire plant is harvested in September at the end of its flowering period. Dr. Christopher advised taking lobelia with a stimulant, especially for pain or spasms. It is best taken as a tincture and can be rubbed into the skin. To overdose will always cause vomiting, which releases excess toxins. The variety with white flowers (inflata) is most often used medicinally.

History and Lore

The herb was smoked by the Native Americans, hence the name Indian tobacco. It was introduced to early nineteenth-century settlers and one famous herbalist of the period, Samuel Thomson, said there was no more powerful herb for relieving serious disease. It was used in conjunction with sweat lodges to purify the body since it produced so much vomiting and sweating. It was believed by the American Indians that if a couple who had been fighting would eat lobelia together, their difficulties would be averted. Throwing some of the herb in front of an approaching storm was used as a spell to stop its approach.

Correspondences

Planet: Saturn
Element: Air
Gender: Female
Sign: Libra

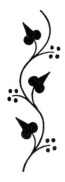

Ma-huang

Ephedra, desert tea, Mormon tea

Ephedra is an American perennial, generally characterized by its leafless, broomlike shrubbery. It has a jointed stem with numerous grooves, and small scalelike leaves growing out of the joints. There are many varieties but it usually has small yellow-green flowers and a seed cone.

Part used: Stems

Therapeutic Profile
Diaphoretic
Anti-inflammatory
Stimulant
Decongestant
Diuretic

Recent Research
Ephedra has demonstrated strong bronchodilatory properties, and is the principle ingredient in several asthma preparations. Research indicates it also has anti-inflammatory and antiallergic activity. It has a thermogenic effect and is a strong central nervous system stimulant.

Medicinal Uses; Catalysts and Combinations
Perhaps the most powerful herbs for the respiratory system are ma-huang and lobelia, but both are very potent and need to be used with some caution. There are many species of ephedra but the Chinese variety (ma-huang) is the one with a concentrated amount of ephedrine, which is the main stimulant and antiasthmatic. It sharpens the mind and stimulates the body. It is useful in treating asthma, emphysema, and colds. It has been used for hay fever and other environmental allergies. It is the dieter's herb because it both reduces hunger and increases metabolism. Ephedra alleviates the pain of arthritis and is useful for treating low blood pressure.

Dosage and Administration
Simmer 1–2 teaspoons of the dried herb in 1½ cups of water for 10 minutes; drink twice a day. In tincture form, take ½ to 1 teaspoon. Powdered capsules are available, usually in combination with other herbs. Do NOT overuse; see precautions in chapter 4.

Gathering and Useful Notes
The young branches should be gathered in the fall before frost, and dried in the sun. The American varieties (Mormon tea) have little ephedrine and therefore little of the stimulant effect. Ma-huang may cause heart palpitations or nervousness. Do not use if you have high blood pressure or diabetes. Do not use with an MAO inhibitor.

History and Lore
There is evidence that the ancient Egyptians used ephedra for irritated throat membranes, and the Chinese have used it to treat asthma for 5,000 years. It was mentioned in the Indian Vedas. The West got it from China, and it was perhaps one of the first imported herbs. The North American Indians made a desert tea from one species of the plant. Its constituents were isolated in 1927 and used as a pharmacologic agent for asthma and hay fever. The early Mormon settlers preferred it to coffee or tea, hence the name "Mormon tea." The synthetic copy of ephedra is epinephrine, and has been used as common street "speed." However, it is difficult to extract from the herb in its natural state.

Correspondences
Planet: Mars
Element: Fire
Gender: Male
Sign: Aries

Marshmallow

Althea, sweet weed

Marshmallow is a perennial that grows two to four feet high, usually in moist meadows. The stems are without branches and woolly. The flowers are usually white, appearing on multiple stalks. The soft leaves are serrated and the root is white and mucilaginous.

Parts used: Root, leaves

Therapeutic Profile
Demulcent
Emollient
Diuretic
Pectoral
Vulnerary

Recent Research
It has been determined that the herb is 35 percent mucilage, and when in contact with water it forms a protective gel with soothing emollient properties.

Medicinal Uses; Catalysts and Combinations
Marshmallow is a mucilaginous herb rich in calcium and pectin. Dr. Christopher believed that it was also a powerful source of oxygen, which is why it has such strong wound-healing properties. It is very healing to any inflamed tissue, external or internal. The combination of its diuretic and demulcent actions make it useful for urinary tract infections or ulcers. It is very healing to stomach tissue and makes a good vaginal douche. Marshmallow is also very soothing for bronchitis and sore throat. It is strengthening to varicose veins and is useful for some allergies. As a poultice, it is excellent for external wounds, bites, or sprains, and has even been used to arrest gangrene. Combine with slippery elm and mullein for sore throat, or with comfrey as a poultice.

Dosage and Administration

Boil 2 teaspoons of the chopped root in 1½ cups water for 10–15 minutes; strain and drink 1 cup several times a day. Or place 2 tablespoons of the leaf and root in 1 cup cold water, let stand several hours, and strain. Fresh roots may also be chewed. Take the tincture, up to 40 drops (or 2–3 capsules), with plenty of water.

Gathering and Useful Notes

Collect leaves in summer after the plant has flowered and dig the root in late autumn. Cut into cross sections and dry. To make a poultice, use 2 ounces each of marshmallow and comfrey, and boil in 2 quarts of water. Soak a towel and use hot; keep body part bound for 1 hour. It can also be mixed with milk and drunk for sore throats.

History and Lore

The ancient Greeks thought marshmallow was one of the most medicinal herbs. Its Greek name, *althea*, means "to cure." It was perhaps first used by Hippocrates for wound healing. In the Bible it is mentioned as a food eaten during famine (Job 30: 3,4). This was undoubtedly useful, since it is such a calcium- and vitamin-rich plant, possessing 286,000 units of vitamin A per pound. At one time it was actually an ingredient in marshmallows and recipes can still be found for using it as a sweet (it would be much more nutritious than the bag of chemicals that passes for marshmallows today). In folklore, it was believed that the plant was sacred, for it attracted good spirits.

Correspondences

Planet: Venus
Element: Water
Gender: Female
Sign: Pisces

Milk Thistle

Mary thistle, silymarin

Milk thistle is a tall, spiny plant that grows wild in many rocky areas. It has a stout, branched stem, and dark green, white-veined leaves with scalloped edges. It is crowned by a large purple flower surrounded by spiny leaflets.

Parts used: Leaves, seeds

Therapeutic Profile
Bitter
Hepatic
Antioxidant
Cholagogue
Demulcent
Nervine

Recent Research
Numerous studies have indicated that the herb protects the liver against specific toxins and it stimulates new liver cells to replace old ones. It exhibits strong antioxidant properties in vitro.

Medicinal Uses; Catalysts and Combinations
This common weed contains some of the most powerful liver-protecting agents known. It protects against poisoning from certain mushrooms, chemicals, and other toxins. The silymarin complex accelerates protein synthesis and stimulates the liver to produce free radical scavengers. It increases immune response and helps eliminate infections. Since the liver is the major site of detoxification, it is good for treating cirrhosis, hepatitis, jaundice, and poisoning. It is strengthening for the kidneys and gallbladder, and has been used successfully with psoriasis. The leaves are used for mild stomach problems. The seeds are potent liver cleaners and are frequently used in detoxification programs. Complementary agents include dandelion, grape seed, pine bark, and turmeric.

Dosage and Administration

The therapeutic substances in milk thistle are not water soluble, so most teas are ineffective. However, some herbalists advise steeping 1 teaspoon of the seeds in 1 cup of water; drink in slow mouthfuls. Or take up to 25 drops of the tincture. In capsule form, 200 milligrams may be taken twice daily.

Gathering and Useful Notes

Gather seed heads (which are armed with needles at the top) when mature and store in a warm place for several days. Then shake and collect the seeds. Milk thistle is harmless even in large doses. It is a valuable tool in the recovery program of alcohol or drug addiction.

History and Lore

There is a legend that the plant got its white-veined leaves from the Virgin Mary, since it resembles mother's milk. The seeds of milk thistle have been used medicinally for more than 2,000 years. The Romans used it as a bile cleanser, one of its most noted properties today. In the Middle Ages, it was considered protection against melancholy. One of the most protective effects in the modern era has been against the severe poisoning of the deathcap mushroom, *Amanita phalloides,* which will prevent death if administered within twenty-four hours. One legend reports that, if worn around the neck as an amulet, the herb will exert a magical influence on snakes. It was considered by the ancients to be the seat of emotions.

Correspondences
  Planet: Jupiter
  Element: Fire
  Gender: Male
  Sign: Sagittarius

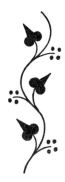

Motherwort

Mother herb, lion's tail

The herb has a square stem, which is erect and slightly purple. Its leaves are rough, dark green, five-lobed, and opposite. The downy flowers are pale purple or white, bell-shaped, and appear in whorls.

Parts used: Flower tops, leaves

Therapeutic Profile

Sedative
Antispasmodic
Diuretic
Cardiotonic
Emmenagogue

Recent Research

The extract of motherwort has been shown to have hypotensive activity. Preparations of motherwort have sedative effects stronger than valerian and may cause paralysis of the central nervous system in large doses.

Medicinal Uses; Catalysts and Combinations

Motherwort has the reputation of being a woman's herb. It is excellent for most menopausal symptoms, including hot flashes, anxiety, insomnia, edema, and depression. It will reduce heart palpitations, relieve constipation, and restore thickness to vaginal walls. It is valuable in delayed or suppressed menstruation, but should be avoided if there is excessive bleeding. Motherwort can also be employed as a douche for vaginitis. The herb is becoming quite famous as a heart tonic, as numerous studies have demonstrated. It promotes circulation, dissolves blood clots, and helps alleviate angina. Use with hawthorn for the heart, and chamomile for nerves.

Dosage and Administration

Pour 1 cup of boiling water over 2 teaspoon of the dried herb; steep 10 minutes. Drink once or twice a day. Or take 10–15 drops of the tincture in a glass of water.

Gathering and Useful Notes

Gather flowering tops in summer after full bloom. A syrup may be made of the extract, since it is very bitter to the taste. Soak 4 ounces of the flowers in cold water for 6 hours, bring to a boil, strain, stir in brown sugar to taste, and store in a cool place. Do not use daily as the sedative properties may become habituating. Do not use if pregnant.

History and Lore

The botanical name (*Leonurus cardiaca*) means "lion hearted" and the herb has long been revered as a faithful heart tonic. In the East, it is associated with longevity in women who take it regularly. Perhaps its calming effects went a long way to alleviate the stress that, in the West, seems to cut life so short. It was used by Chinese courtesans to prevent pregnancy. The early colonists used it as an aid in expelling afterbirth. It is thought that drinking motherwort before bedtime will eliminate nightmares. It also gives one a sense of purpose, and direction in one's life's work.

Correspondences

   Planet: Sun
   Element: Fire
   Gender: Female
   Sign: Leo

Mugwort

Felon herb, Artemis herb, artemisia

Mugwort is a common perennial with a downy, slightly grooved stem. It has alternate leaf stems with branching leaflets, downy white on the underside, very linear and coarsely toothed. Flower heads are spiked and reddish-brown or yellow.

Parts used: Root, leaves

Therapeutic Profile
Cholagogue
Emmenagogue
Diaphoretic
Nervine
Bitter

Recent Research
There is not as much research on mugwort as motherwort, although it has some of the same herbal effects in treating amenorrhea.

Medicinal Uses; Catalysts and Combinations
Mugwort leaves are used to stimulate late menstrual flow and also in easing cramps. It can be used for digestive stimulation and is soothing for stomach disorders. It is a mild nervine for easing anxiety, and has been used for insomnia. The Chinese technique of moxabustion helps to promote blood circulation, relax the underlying nerves, and stimulate the immune system. Mugwort will stimulate the gallbladder and aid in eliminating toxins through perspiration. Complementary agents include black cohosh and motherwort.

Dosage and Administration

Steep 2 tablespoons of the dried herb in 1 pint of water for 20 minutes, drink several times a day. Or take 5–20 drops of the tincture. Prepared capsules are available.

Gathering and Useful Notes

Gather flowering tops in late summer when in full bloom. Mugwort can be burned and the ash used topically for bleeding. The leaves have a cotton consistency and are used to make "moxas," a Chinese herbal stick burned into the skin in place of needles. Or make a hot fomentation from the tea, wrung out on a towel. Apply for cramps.

History and Lore

Mugwort was used by Native Americans for flu or fever. They also used it ritually in smudging: it was believed to purify the air and cleanse the negative spirits. According to ancient folklore, one cannot be harmed by wild beasts if wearing mugwort. The Chinese, too, used it as an herb of protection, hanging it over their doors to banish evil demons. It was sacred to witches, who used it to wash their magic crystal balls. Like motherwort, mugwort is good for dreaming; a pillow stuffed with the herb will bring prophetic dreams, which should be recorded at soon as possible upon awakening. One legend tells us that St. John the Baptist wore a girdle of mugwort to sustain him in the desert.

Correspondences

Planet: Venus
Element: Earth
Gender: Female
Sign: Taurus

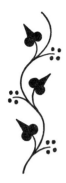

Mullein

Jacob's staff, velvet plant, feltwort

Mullein grows about two feet high in many pastures in North America. It has a stout wooly felt stem and the leaves are also thickly white-felted. They are gray-green, large, and pointed, forming a rosette at the base of the stem. Yellow flowers grow in cylindrical spikes.

Parts used: Leaves, flowers, root

Therapeutic Profile

Antispasmodic
Demulcent
Diuretic
Expectorant
Pectoral
Vulnerary
Emollient

Recent Research

Mullein has been shown to provide a thick mucilaginous coating to membranes, thus aiding in inhibiting the absorption of allergens.

Medicinal Uses; Catalysts and Combinations

Mullein leaf has been used in a variety of respiratory problems, from a simple cough to emphysema and asthma. It may be smoked for bronchial congestion. Jethro Kloss, in *Back to Eden,* advises burning the root and inhaling the fumes for asthma. The oil is a remedy for earache. A fomentation of one variety, black mullein, is effective for the pain and swelling of hemorrhoids. The root can be used for cramps and diarrhea. A poultice of the freshly crushed flowers has been used to eliminate warts. Use with marshmallow and lobelia for respiratory problems.

Dosage and Administration

Pour 1 cup of boiling water over 2 teaspoon of the dried leaves; steep 10 minutes. Drink 3 times a day. Or take 10–30 drops of the tincture. The oil is also commercially available for earaches.

Gathering and Useful Notes

Clip leaves in summer before they turn brown, and dry in the shade. Gather flowers in early fall and carefully avoid any moisture when drying. A fomentation may be made from mullein and lobelia leaves: Simmer 1 ounce of each in 2 quarts of water, and apply as hot as possible. You can make your own oil by mixing the flowers with olive oil and leaving in the sun for seven days, shaking frequently, then draining the oil.

History and Lore

Mullein has an interesting fatty matter that was noticed by Dioscorides to be effective against swelling and pain. It was a favorite herb of numerous Native American tribes. During the Civil War, the Confederates used it frequently for respiratory disorders. In India, it was first used against certain bacteria and was eventually discovered to be effective against tuberculosis. It has numerous other practical applications, including using the stems as candle wicks. The stalks were sometimes dipped in suet and the torches burned at funerals. It was a favorite plant for drying and smoking. Witches were said to burn it while making incantations. In folklore, it was believed to instill courage if worn, or to obtain love if carried.

Correspondences

Planet: Jupiter
Element: Fire
Gender: Female
Sign: Sagittarius

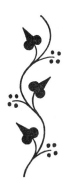

Myrrh

Gum myrrh, karan, myrrha

The myrrh tree grows only about ten feet high, with a thick trunk, sharp spines, and white-gray bark. The leaves are trifoliate; the fruit is pea-sized; and the gum, or resin, is a reddish brown.

Part used: Resin

Therapeutic Profile
Antiseptic
Antibiotic
Astringent
Carminative
Expectorant
Vulnerary
Antifungal

Recent Research
The antimicrobial and disinfectant properties of the herb have been documented in both America and China. It appears to increase white blood cells and also to strengthen capillary activity.

Medicinal Uses; Catalysts and Combinations
Myrrh is a strong antimicrobial herb used to treat a variety of infections. It has long been found effective for ulcers of the mouth, gingivitis, and pyorrhea. The herb can be used as a gargle and it sweetens the breath also. It is an excellent antiseptic for open wounds. It has antifungal activity for some ear infections and has been used for candida yeast. Chronic sinus and bronchial congestions have improved with the administration of the herb. A salve can be made for hemorrhoids and sores. It will expel worms when combined with cayenne. Use with goldenseal, echinacea, and garlic for infections.

Dosage and Administration

Steep 1 teaspoon powdered herb and 1 teaspoon raspberry in 1 pint of hot water; use as a mouthwash. It may also be drunk, 1–3 cups a day. Or take ½ teaspoon of the tincture in a glass of water.

Gathering and Useful Notes

The myrrh sap exudes naturally from the bark, drying as it gets older and harder. To purify the breath, mix 1 teaspoon each of myrrh and goldenseal powders, steep 10 minutes in 1 pint of boiling water, pour off the liquid, and sip several times a day. Do not take myrrh for more than two weeks.

History and Lore

Myrrh is mentioned many times in the Bible and is considered a very sacred herb to the Kabbalists, where it belongs to Binah, the Almighty Mother, who is the Eternal Sea. She is sometimes called Bitter (mara) Sea. The ancient Greeks believed the resin drops were from Myrrha, who was changed into a myrrh tree to escape the wrath of Aphrodite. Myrrh was part of the embalming mixture of the Egyptians, who considered it to be aromatic and sacred. It was burned in the temples of both Ra and Isis. The incense is generally associated with purifying a space and instilling a sense of peace. It is often added to other incense mixtures to potentate the effects. The Hebrews used it to anoint the tabernacle and the ark, and its holiness was associated with Jesus at the birth of the Christian era.

Correspondences

Planet: Saturn
Element: Water
Gender: Female
Sign: Capricorn

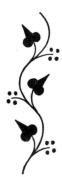

Oatstraw

Groats, oats

One of the most popular edible grains, oatstraw is an annual grass with a jointed stem growing about two to four feet high. It has narrow, green, flat leaves, a fibrous root, and delicate two-flowered spikes.

Parts used: Straw, grain

Therapeutic Profile
Nervine
Demulcent
Vulnerary
Antispasmodic
Cardiotonic
Nutritive

Recent Research
It has been determined by scientists in Israel that oatstraw has estrogenic activity. Oat bran has lowered cholesterol in a number of tests.

Medicinal Uses; Catalysts and Combinations
Oatstraw has been found very useful for menopausal women, not only offering a calming effect on the nerves but also enriching the bones with a dense form of natural calcium. It is a nutritive herb with other minerals as well, and is particularly nourishing for the pancreas, liver, adrenals, blood vessels, and nerves. Oatstraw is used for depression as well as anxiety. The herb helps to stabilize blood sugar levels, reduces cholesterol, and improves circulatory functioning. Oats are a very nutritious and easily digested food for the elderly or convalescing. It is an excellent overall tonic. Combine with skullcap and Saint John's Wort for change-of-life depression.

Dosage and Administration

Pour boiling water over 2 teaspoons of the dried grass and steep 10 minutes; drink 3 times daily. Or take 10–20 drops of the extract. Oats may be taken freely as an edible grain.

Gathering and Useful Notes

Gather the straw and grain in late August; hang the stalks to dry. A relaxing bath is made by taking a pound of the shredded grass and boiling in 2 quarts of water, draining after 20 minutes, and adding to bath water. For healthy skin, tie rolled oats in cheesecloth and rub on the body while bathing.

History and Lore

In folklore, the oat plant was believed to attract prosperity. Oatstraw was thought to restore regenerative powers and make the brain sharper. This may be based in some fact, since the herb is so rich in silicon, which is reputed to have an effect on the cerebral cortex, the part of the brain that thinks and observes. The English did not believe that the oat plant was good for anything except feeding to horses. The Scottish, with their good sense, taught them otherwise. Oats now are regarded as one of the most healthy modern foods, and it also makes a popular facial mask. It has been a primary food source for many cultures for centuries. Some herbalists advise using the flower essence to discern clarity about life direction.

Correspondences

Planet: Venus
Element: Air
Gender: Female
Sign: Libra

Oregon Grape

Grape root, mountain grape

Oregon grape is an evergreen common to mountain slopes. It has branched stems about three feet long and alternate, toothed, shiny leaves. The flowers are small and yellow-green, and it has blue-purple berries. The root is knotty, tough, and tubular.

Part used: Root

Therapeutic Profile
Alternative
Cholagogue
Laxative
Tonic
Antibiotic
Diuretic
Hepatic

Recent Research
Laboratory studies indicate that Oregon grape has impressive antibacterial activity.

Medicinal Uses; Catalysts and Combinations
Oregon grape has long been considered one of the finest blood purifiers; that is, it is an excellent tonic for the liver and is targeted specifically for skin problems. It is useful for psoriasis and eczema. It has been used as a mild laxative, or is combined with other herbs in a laxative formula. It is useful for stomach and gallbladder conditions, and is especially soothing for nausea. In the past, it was part of a treatment for syphilis, jaundice, and Crohn's disease. The herb is antiseptic to the kidneys and to the vaginal tissue when it is used as a douche. It is rich in iron and effective in treating anemia. It is advised

for menstrual irregularities. Combine with garlic, echinacea, and goldenseal as a natural antibiotic.

Dosage and Administration
Simmer 2 teaspoons of the dried root in 1 cup of water for 10 minutes. Drink 3 times a day. Or take 10–30 drops of the tincture, or 1–3 grams of the powder.

Gathering and Useful Notes
Collect roots in late fall, and slice to dry. A strong tea can be made of the chopped root and used externally as a fomentation. It is also available in homeopathic therapy for skin problems and herpes. In most cases, it may be substituted for goldenseal, since its therapeutic actions are nearly the same, and use of it as a substitute is an ecological way to preserve the now-threatened goldenseal root.

History and Lore
Oregon grape is a favorite medicinal plant in the Pacific Northwest, and the state flower of Oregon. Its counterpart is barberry, which grows in the Northeast. The shrub was introduced to England from America in the early 1800s. In the Spanish-American tradition it was called "herb of the blood." It was a much-revered tonic in the early West, and was believed to keep the skin looking ever-youthful. It was overharvested and almost exterminated. In folklore, it was thought that to wear the root would make one popular. Oregon grape is not to be confused with grape seed, a food supplement that has been growing in popularity for its impressive antioxidant properties. (See pine bark for more information on pycnogenol products.)

Correspondences
   Planet: Mars
   Element: Earth
   Gender: Male
   Sign: Capricorn

Pau d'Arco

Taheebo, lapacho

The lapacho tree is found in the rainforests of South America. It is an evergreen with broad leaves and scarlet or purple flowers. The bark and inner wood is extremely hard and slow to decay.

Part used: Bark

Therapeutic Profile

Alternative
Immunostimulant
Hepatic
Bitter
Tonic
Anti-inflammatory
Antitumor
Antibiotic
Antifungal

Recent Research

There is much scientific interest in the herb as a parasiticide and an antitumor and antifungal treatment. It is one of the most important plants in cancer research.

Medicinal Uses; Catalysts and Combinations

Although new to the West, Pau d'Arco has long been considered a "miracle" plant in South America for its many medicinal properties. It is an effective antibiotic and antiviral herb, and has been tested numerous times for its healing activity for malignancies, especially leukemia. Its anti-inflammatory activity helps to eliminate pain, and it is a powerful curative for ulcers, diabetes, arthritis, ringworm, eczema, anemia, urinary tract infections, and candida. It is very rich in iron and an excellent blood purifier. As a general immune strengthener, use with echinacea, garlic, goldenseal, and milk thistle.

Dosage and Administration
Simmer 1 ounce of the bark in 1 pint of water. Drink ½ to 1 cup 2 or 3 times a day, or take 30–40 drops of the tincture. Commercial capsules are available; follow the dosage on the bottle.

Gathering and Useful Notes
The inner bark of the tree is what is most effective and should be stripped carefully, since the outer bark, which is often sold as pau d' arco, contains little of the healing properties. It should also be aged. A vaginal douche can be made from the tea. It may also be applied to the skin.

History and Lore
The native Indians of the South American rainforests have used lapacho for thousands of years, even prior to the Inca civilization. It has long been thought of as a general tonic for nearly everything, similar to ginseng in the East. Lapacho, which is the Indian name of the plant, means "the divine tree." It was first discovered as a useful anti-cancer agent by U.S. physicians in the 1960s, but research is proceeding much slower than in the southern hemisphere, where it is a standard form of treatment for certain kinds of cancer (blood and skin). It was noticed by the natives that the tree never attracted mold or mildew after being chopped down (hence its antifungal properties) and is known as the tree with strength and vigor.

Correspondences
    Planet: Jupiter
    Element: Fire
    Gender: Male
    Sign: Sagittarius

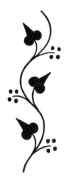

Pennyroyal

European pennyroyal, fleabane

The herb has two varieties, but the one from Europe (*Mentha pulegium*) is a ground-hugging mint with a square stem. Only the violet flower stalk rises above ground. It has opposite egg-shaped leaves and light brown seeds.

Parts used: Leaves, flowers

Therapeutic Profile
Diaphoretic
Emmenagogue
Antispasmodic
Carminative
Antiseptic
Febrifuge
Nervine

Recent Research
Pennyroyal extracts have been shown to stimulate the uterus in several experimental studies.

Medicinal Uses; Catalysts and Combinations
Pennyroyal is used to treat lung problems, and is effective for colds and flu. It is a strong promoter of menstruation, and may also induce abortions, so it should be avoided during pregnancy. It has caused death when taken in very large doses. The oil has long been used as an insect repellent. It may be used as an herbal pet flea collar. Pennyroyal is helpful in expelling gas. The volatile oil acts as a carminative and soothes the stomach. It has a calming effect on the nerves. It promotes perspiration and is useful in treating circulation problems. Combine with chamomile.

Dosage and Administration
Use 1 teaspoon of the herb with 1 cup of water. Drink 2–3 cups a day. Or take up to 40 drops of the tincture. Avoid ingesting the oil.

Gathering and Useful Notes
The herb should be gathered just before it flowers, usually in late July. Hang to dry. Use carefully; there are dangers of death from self-induced abortions. Use the dry herb; the oil should only be used externally. Discontinue if the herb causes diarrhea.

History and Lore
Pennyroyal was a popular herb in the Roman world as an insect repellent, since it was noticed that the aromatic properties repelled fleas. Hence the name "fleabane." The Greek doctor Dioscorides added the important therapeutic information that it promotes menses and it was used to help expel afterbirth. The North American Indians used it as a calming agent. It is safe when taken in the herb form, but it was discovered that the oil was very dangerous in the late 1800s, when the first death was reported. It would take many gallons of the tea to be as toxic as two tablespoons of the oil, which was reported to cause death in one medical journal. In folklore, penny-royal was thought to restore peace to quarreling couples, and was carried for protection during travel.

Correspondences
Planet: Mars
Element: Earth
Gender: Female
Sign: Capricorn

Peppermint

Balm mint, lamb mint

Peppermint has a square stem and is the most pungent of all the mints. It has shining, serrated leaves, and tiny purple flowers.

Part used: Leaves

Therapeutic Profile

Carminative
Diaphoretic
Anti-emetic
Nervine
Antiseptic
Anti-inflammatory

Recent Research

Studies indicate that the mint normalizes gastrointestinal activity, possesses anti-ulcer and anti-inflammatory properties, and is effective against several kinds of bacteria.

Medicinal Uses; Catalysts and Combinations

Peppermint is one of the most effective agents for stomach problems in the herbal kingdom. It relieves gas and is excellent for nausea and diarrhea. The mint is very useful for travel sickness and vomiting during pregnancy. Its essential oils stimulate the gallbladder and encourage bile secretion. It has a relaxing effect on the whole system and is good for spasms and convulsions, even in small children. The oil is used in many mouthwashes and toothpastes, and is antibacterial as well as pleasantly aromatic. It is useful in treating fevers, colds, and flu. It eases the tension and anxiety connected with headaches, and externally may be used for skin inflammations. Peppermint makes a wonderful flavoring agent. Combine with boneset and yarrow for flu.

Dosage and Administration
Pour 1 cup of boiling water over 1 teaspoon of the dried herb and steep 10 minutes. Drink as often as desired. Five to fifteen drops per cup of the oil can also be added to hot water. Or take 1–2 teaspoons of the tincture.

Gathering and Useful Notes
The plant should be harvested right before flowering, and hung to dry. It can also be used fresh. Both the herb and the oil can be used freely, and are very safe. The oil makes a pleasant and relaxing massage oil. Rub on temples for headache. However, do not apply oil directly to the face, especially children's.

History and Lore
Peppermint has been a common folk medicine in many Indian tribes in both North and South America. It was valued as a form of payment for taxes in the ancient Near East. Mint is sacred to the Greek goddess Mintha, who was changed by Persephone into the herb when caught in a love affair with her husband Pluto. It was used in wreaths at Roman initiations. In folklore, it is believed that it cleanses a home of negativity if rubbed on the furniture and floors. It is also placed under a pillow to induce relaxing sleep and dreams. It has long been used as a calming agent and in one study of university students it was effective in alleviating the anxiety associated with test-taking skills.

Correspondences
Planet: Venus
Element: Water
Gender: Female
Sign: Pisces

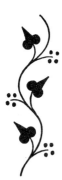

$\mathcal{P}$ine Bark

Anneda tree, Maritime pine, pycnogenol

Maritime pine grows abundantly along the coasts of southern France. It has thick clumps of evergreen needles and a deep reddish-brown bark, with a long, fairly smooth pine cone.

Parts used: Bark, needles

Therapeutic Profile
Immunostimulant
Antioxidant
Anti-inflammatory
Adaptogen
Antitumor
Cardiotonic
Stimulant

Recent Research

There have been a great number of studies testing pycnogenol. It stops free radical damage in vitro and in vivo, and is twenty times more effective than vitamin C. It greatly strengthens blood vessels and inhibits tumor production.

Medicinal Uses; Catalysts and Combinations

The ingredient isolated from pine bark (and also grape seed) that constitutes its principle "magic" are the proanthocyanidins. Pine bark has been found to be an excellent defender of the circulatory system. It prevents blood clots and helps lower cholesterol. The herb has been used in Europe for two decades to strengthen blood vessels, reduce edema, and arrest varicose veins. Pycnogenol will improve the elasticity and appearance of the skin. It protects the body from arthritis and cancer by building a strong immune system. It has been prescribed for diabetic retinopathy, hay fever, inflammations, and sports injuries. Combine with garlic, algae, and hawthorn as a daily antioxidant.

Dosage and Administration
The medicinal actions from either pine bark or grape seed are generally not available in tea form. Capsules or tablets usually come in 30–50 milligram concentrates. Take as freely as needed, up to about 150 milligrams a day.

Gathering and Useful Notes
Although the pycnogenol from pine bark can be harvested and extracted in a number of places where pine grows, the patented commercial source is the bark of the European coastal pine. Some researchers say it should be 85 percent distilled concentrate of the extract in order to be effective as a highly bioactive antioxidant. Studies demonstrate it is well tolerated and safe even in large doses.

History and Lore
The pine tree has a rich, legendary history. The pine was sacred to many of the gods in the ancient world: Pan, Venus, Poseidon, Dionysus, Attis, Cybele, and Jupiter. Pine cones represented fertility as well as a healthy old age. Pine needles were burned as an aid in cleansing a home of evil vibrations. They were believed to reverse curses. The incense was used in rituals to attract money. It was offered to the god of the sea, Poseidon, before embarking on a journey by water. The pitch of the tree was used to caulk the boat. In Japan, a pine branch was placed over the door of a home for good luck. In the sixteenth century its nutritional value was revealed to the French explorer Jacques Cartier, who was told by an old Indian to make a tea of the bark and give it to his crew, then dying of scurvy. The tea saved their lives.

Correspondences
   Planet: Mars
   Element: Water
   Gender: Male
   Sign: Scorpio

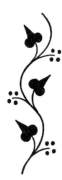

$\mathcal{P}$lantain

Ribgrass, cuckoo's bread, waybread

Plantain grows up to eighteen inches high, with a stiff, smooth stem and long, broad, lanceolate leaves that are very dark green. It has dense spikes of purple-brown flowers divided into four leaflets.

Parts used: Whole plant

Therapeutic Profile
Alternative
Astringent
Antiseptic
Diuretic
Emollient
Vulnerary
Febrifuge
Hemostatic
Expectorant
Demulcent

Recent Research
Research indicates that plantain is effective against skin dermatitis and obesity. New studies demonstrate that it prevents absorption of lipids, aiding in cholesterol regulation.

Medicinal Uses; Catalysts and Combinations
Plantain is a useful herb for cough irritations, hoarseness, and mucous congestion. It is good for urinary tract infections, and its diuretic properties help to rid the body of poisons. It also absorbs toxins from the bowel. Its soothing demulcent qualities make it excellent for gastritis and all irritated internal membranes. It has been used for hemorrhoids and skin inflammations. A poultice of the herb is effective in the treatment of poison oak and poison ivy. It also acts to

curb bleeding of wounds. The oil is also helpful for vaginal itching or burning. Combine with burdock.

Dosage and Administration
Pour 1 cup of boiling water over 2 teaspoons of the dried herb; steep 10 minutes. Or take 1 teaspoon of the fluid extract 2–3 times daily. Powdered capsules may be taken; follow the directions on the bottle.

Gathering and Useful Notes
Harvest the herb throughout the summer and dry in the hot sun, quickly, if possible. Make sure the leaves are mature. An ointment can be made by simmering the mashed herb slowly in olive oil for about an hour. The fresh leaves can also be pounded into a paste and applied to wounds.

History and Lore
Plantain was a favorite herb of the early colonists in treating wounds and skin diseases. The English called plantain "all-heal," and to the American Indians it was known as "life medicine." It was believed to repel snakes and instill strength. In folklore, it was carried for protection or hung in homes to protect from evil spirits. In medieval Christian art, it was a symbol of the path to Christ. In another symbolic motif, it represented a maiden who waited so long near the roadside for her lover that she eventually turned into the roadside herb. Dr. Christopher believed that it was the greatest herb for blood poisoning, and cured several people of serious poisonings and possible amputations by applying his "magical" plantain poultices.

Correspondences
Planet: Venus
Element: Earth
Gender: Female
Sign: Taurus

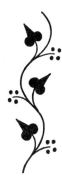

Prickly Ash

Toothache bark, angelica tree

Prickly ash is a shrub that grows up to twenty feet high, with branches that bear thorns that are quite large. The leaves are alternate and hairy and the flowers a pale yellow-green that appear in small clusters before the leaves. The fruit is a small berry with black seeds.

Parts used: Bark, fruit

Therapeutic Profile
Alternative
Astringent
Antiseptic
Diaphoretic
Nervine
Rubefacient
Expectorant

Recent Research
There is little research in the herb, but the Merck Index reports that prickly ash possesses a constituent called asarinin, which has anti-tubercular properties.

Medicinal Uses; Catalysts and Combinations
The herb has long been viewed as an effective panacea, good for most everything. It increases circulation and eases leg cramps and varicose veins. Externally, it has a calming effect on the nervous system and has been used to treat rheumatism. It is an effective expectorant and is added to many cold remedies. The herb will cause a numbing sensation in the mouth and has been used in the relief of toothaches. Its antiseptic properties make it also useful as tooth powder. It is effective for cramps and fevers. Externally, it may be applied as a poultice for wounds. Use with sarsaparilla and black cohosh for arthritic pains.

Dosage and Administration
Boil 1 teaspoon of the dried bark in 1 cup of water. Drink 1–2 cups a day, cold. Or take 10–20 drops of the tincture.

Gathering and Useful Notes
Collect the berries in late summer and strip the bark from the stems before drying. Prickly ash has been used to treat pyorrhea, and a tooth powder can be made by mixing the herb with myrrh and bayberry; ground the powders together and brush when there are gum problems.

History and Lore
Prickly ash gained notoriety in America in the mid-nineteenth century during the outbreak of Asian cholera. American Indians also used it to treat colds and toothaches; they christened it the "toothache tree." It is considered by some alternative therapists to be a useful aid in the fight against cancer, and has been used as a principle ingredient in the Hoxsey formulas. Harry Hoxsey began prescribing the famous Hoxsey Cancer Formula in the 1930s and, by the 1950s, had founded clinics in seventeen states. The FDA closed the cancer clinics but the formula is still available in Mexico. In folklore the berries were collected for use in love spells. There are many reports of an electric feeling upon ingestion of the tea.

Correspondences
    Planet: Mars
    Element: Fire
    Gender: Male
    Sign: Aries

Queen of the Meadow

Gravel root, kidney root

The plant is a North American perennial common to meadows. It has a hollow stem and grows up to ten feet high, with a woody, fibrous root and coarsely serrated leaves. The flowers are purple or white and grow in loose clusters.

Parts used: Root, flowers, leaves

Therapeutic Profile
Diuretic
Astringent
Tonic
Nervine
Anti-inflammatory

Recent Research
In clinical trials, the herb has been shown effective for most forms of inflammatory stress. It also prevents the precipitation of uric acid crystals.

Medicinal Uses; Catalysts and Combinations
Queen of the Meadow is used principally as a diuretic and is an effective agent against kidney stones, cystitis, and urethritis. It is especially useful for the more chronic conditions. It is a good overall tonic for the kidneys, bladder, liver, prostate, and uterus. It has been used for edema and lower back pain. Its calming activity makes it a reliable herb for women during menstruation, combined with its activity of toning the female organs and pelvic muscles. It is a well-known aid for the pain of rheumatism and gout. Use with marshmallow and uva ursi for kidney complaints. It also combines well with goldenseal or Oregon grape.

Dosage and Administration
Simmer 1 teaspoon of the roots and herb in 1½ cups of water for 10 minutes. Drink several times a day. Or take 1 teaspoon of the tincture 3 times daily.

Gathering and Useful Notes
Dig roots in autumn after the herb has flowered, and slice to dry. Dr. Christopher advises drinking a weak tea mixed with tofu milk frequently. He also advises soaking the root for two hours before boiling.

History and Lore
Queen of the Meadow was used by some North American tribes as an aphrodisiac. One legend tells the story of a famous New England Indian by the name of Joe Pye who gained notoriety by curing typhus with the herb, and in some places it was known as "joe pye weed." One of the more famous Dr. Christopher formulas incorporated it as a primary herb in the treatment of the prostate, which saved many grateful men from operations.

Correspondences
  Planet: Saturn
  Element: Water
  Gender: Female
  Sign: Libra

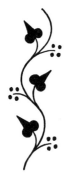

Raspberry

Red raspberry, bramble

The plant is erect and has many spiny branches with prickles. The leaves are ovate, come in pairs with serrated margins, and are hairy and pale green. It has small white flower clusters and red succulent berries.

Parts used: Leaves, berries

Therapeutic Profile

Astringent
Tonic
Alternative
Antispasmodic
Emmenagogue
Anti-emetic

Recent Research

Research indicates that the herb relaxes the smooth muscles of the uterus and intestine.

Medicinal Uses; Catalysts and Combinations

Red raspberry is the most famous plant in the herb kingdom for protecting young mothers during pregnancy. It has been used to ease morning sickness and is good for nausea in general. It is an excellent uterine tonic and helps strengthen the stomach, bowels, and all internal tissue. It is useful in easing the pains of delivery and is one of the richest herbs in mineral nutrients, especially iron and manganese. It prevents hemorrhaging and false labor. Not only is the herb a favorite for pregnant women, it is also effective in treating colic, colds, diarrhea, fevers, cankerous sores, and bleeding gums in children. Use with licorice, dong quai, or wild yam.

Dosage and Administration

Pour a cup of boiling water over 1 teaspoon of the dried leaves. Drink as often as desired. Take 1 teaspoon of the tincture or powdered capsules; follow the directions on the bottle.

Gathering and Useful Notes

The leaves may be gathered all during the summer, and should be dried slowly. A healing douche may be made of the tea mixed with a little myrrh powder.

History and Lore

Red raspberry has been a popular fruit for at least 2,000 years, but its medicinal properties have gone unnoticed. It was first cultivated in Europe about 400 years ago, and cultivation rapidly spread to England and then to the United States. By the mid-nineteenth century, it was produced as an important crop in the state of Pennsylvania, where several varieties were developed. It has become a favorite herb of pregnant women, and in folklore, it was believed that to carry it would lead to an easy delivery. It was also thought to be an important magical herb for deaths, as a raspberry hung over the doorway keeps the spirit from being confused and attempting to reenter the home.

Correspondences

  Planet: Venus
  Element: Water
  Gender: Female
  Sign: Pisces

Red Clover

Wild clover, trefoil

Clover is a common meadow plant with reddish stems and oval leaves, three to a stem. It has rose-purple flowers in crowded tubular corollas, and is very aromatic.

Part used: Flowers

Therapeutic Profile
Alternative
Antioxidant
Nutritive
Sedative
Antibiotic
Expectorant
Antispasmodic
Diuretic

Recent Research
It has been discovered that an extract of red clover is a strong carcinogenic inhibitor. Antibiotic tests demonstrate its effectiveness against several kinds of bacteria.

Medicinal Uses; Catalysts and Combinations
Red clover is a popular herb in traditional folk medicine and holds much promise in new research. It has been used to stimulate liver and gallbladder activity, and is excellent for skin diseases. It is effective for bronchitis and spasmodic affections. It is soothing to the nerves and is a powerful nutritive herb. It is used by some as an adjunct to cancer treatment, and was one of the ingredients in the famous Hoxsey formula. Studies indicate it has antioxidant activity, and it has been shown to be useful as an antiviral and antimicrobial agent. Use with chaparral and astragalus for rebuilding the immune system.

Dosage and Administration

Steep 2 teaspoons of the flower tops in 1 cup of water for 10 minutes; drink 3–4 times a day. Or take 20 drops of the tincture. Capsules are available, take as directed on bottle.

Gathering and Useful Notes

The flower buds may be collected all summer, although they should be fully bloomed. Clover works best when combined with other alternative herbs. A strong tea can be made as a wash for scaly skin. The fresh flowers can be used to make vinegar.

History and Lore

The herb held a mystical fascination for the ancient Greeks and Romans, and has long been used as an amulet against witchcraft. It was considered the perfect symbol for the Trinity by early Christian missionaries, and the trefoil was kept in the home for protection. The four-leaf clover was thought to bring sure success, and a two-leaf symbolized the affection of lovers. In the late nineteenth century it was a major ingredient in the famous anticancer formula called the Trifolium Compounds. Red clover is an herb that sends its roots deep into the earth; therefore, it has long been used as an important plant food by grazing animals. For the past century its nutritive properties have not gone unnoticed by perceptive herbalists.

Correspondences

Planet: Mercury
Element: Air
Gender: Male
Sign: Gemini

Rose Hips

Dog rose, Japanese rose

The genus *Rosa* are prickly shrubs of many varieties that have trailing or climbing stems and alternate leaves, saw-toothed, with three to five leaflets. The flower comes in many shades and are five-petaled in the wild. The rose hip is the heart of the rose; small, round, and fleshy.

Part used: Hip

Therapeutic Profile

Antiseptic
Nutritive
Tonic
Antioxidant
Antibiotic
Astringent

Recent Research

The rose hip contains compounds that have been proven to contain high amounts of vitamin C, which gives the herb its potent antibiotic and antioxidant properties. Much research has been done with both vitamin C and the bioflavonoids, also a valuable ingredient in rose hips.

Medicinal Uses; Catalysts and Combinations

Rose hips are an excellent tonic to help build the body's defenses against infection. There is sixty times more vitamin C in rose hips than in citrus. Several modern illnesses can benefit from vitamin C, including arteriosclerosis, stress, and suppressed immune function. It is good for general debility, tissue and cartilage strengthening, bladder infections, and fevers. The bioflavonoid properties make it an effective estrogenic agent and it is therefore helpful for PMS and menopause. Complementary agents include cayenne, garlic, and rosemary.

Dosage and Administration
Pour 1 cup of water over 2 teaspoons of cut rose hips, bring to a boil, and simmer several minutes. Or take 1 teaspoon of the tincture as needed. Many vitamin C preparations contain natural rose hips, but not in very high properties.

Gathering and Useful Notes
Gather rose hips in the fall. Dry in the shade and store in a tight container. They will make a delightful tea all winter. There are many varieties of roses, but the best for rose hips are the dog rose (*Rosa canina*) and the Japanese (*Rugosa thunb*). Rose hip syrup is an excellent infection-fighter for children.

History and Lore
Rose hips and petals were frequently used in nineteenth-century pharmaceuticals, often combined with other herbal compounds. Roses have had an association with the numinous, however, much further back than that. The Egyptians considered the oil to be sacred. To the Greeks, it was a plant that belonged to Aphrodite. The medicinal properties were thought to be introduced from Damascus by a crusader. In the Middle Ages it was adapted as the national flower in Britain. The herbalist and saint Hildegard of Bingen recommended rose hip tea as a panacea for many illnesses. In Jungian symbolism, roses represent the selflessness of love and are associated with the heart (the ability to love and nurture). Numerous Christian visionaries have claimed to see the Blessed Virgin Mary's rose garden in Heaven.

Correspondences
   Planet: Venus
   Element: Earth
   Gender: Female
   Sign: Taurus

Rosemary

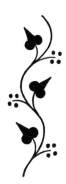

Sea dew, compass weed

Rosemary grows up to five feet high, with a square, brown, woody stem and long, thin, dark green leaves that are very pointed. The flower is pale blue, two-lipped, and tubular.

Parts used: Leaves, flower tops

Therapeutic Profile
Antispasmodic
Aromatic
Carminative
Antiseptic
Cholagogue
Stimulant

Recent Research
One herbal activity recently discovered in an extract of rosemary is its potential as a chemopreventive agent. Hypotensive activity has also been observed in some studies.

Medicinal Uses; Catalysts and Combinations
Rosemary has a calming effect on the digestive system and will ease stomach cramps. It has been used to strengthen the heart and reduce blood pressure. Its antiseptic properties make it useful as a mouthwash. Used externally, it is good for the pains of neuralgia and sciatica. It has a stimulating effect on the liver and also stimulates blood circulation. Rosemary contains constituents that act as an infection fighter and helps to prevent bacteria when applied to wounds. It is good for colds when combined with garlic and rose hips, but should not be used continuously when taken internally.

Dosage and Administration

Use 1–2 teaspoons of the dried herb to 1 cup of hot water; steep 10 minutes. It may be taken 2–3 times a day for colds or stomach upset. Or take 5–10 drops of the tincture. Use capsules in combination with other herbs, not alone.

Gathering and Useful Notes

Gather leaves and flower tops late in summer and hang to dry. The oil is excellent when mixed with olive oil for massage. The aromatic properties make it a delightful addition to potpourris or incenses. When added to shampoo, it will slightly darken the hair, and its astringency makes it a useful addition to skin lotions. It is toxic in large doses internally.

History and Lore

The name "sea dew" is derived from the Latin *ros* and *maris*, and first comes from the Mediterranean coastlands. In the ancient world, it was associated with long memory and restful sleep. It was often cast upon coffins as a symbol of remembrance of the departed. Hung on porches, it was supposed to keep thieves away. It was believed that the fumes promoted healing when burned by the bedside in a sickroom. Rosemary was often woven into a bride's wreath and was a symbol of fidelity. In some South American countries it is frequently used as an insect repellent.

Correspondences

Planet: Sun
Element: Fire
Gender: Male
Sign: Leo

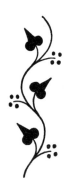

Rue

Herb of grace, garden rue

The herb is a lovely garden plant with a woody stem, bluish shoots, and lacy evergreen leaves. The flowers are bright yellow or yellow-green with wavy petals in loose clusters.

Parts used: All of the parts above ground

Therapeutic Profile

Antispasmodic
Emmenagogue
Stimulant
Bitter
Rubefacient
Cholagogue
Vermifuge

Recent Research

In animal experiments, rue causes strong uterine stimulation, and the extract acts as an abortive agent.

Medicinal Uses; Catalysts and Combinations

Rue has long been used to treat nervous spasms, cramps, and strained muscles. It increases circulation and the oil has been used to ease arthritic and sciatic pains. The tea has been used to expel worms and to promote menstruation. It will relieve griping and other stomach cramps, and has been useful in the treatment of tension headaches. Externally it has been used to remove warts and pimples. It is an abortifacient in large doses and can be very poisonous. Its antiseptic properties make is a good eyewash and gargle. In small doses, combine with pennyroyal to suppress excessive menstruation.

Dosage and Administration
Steep 1 tablespoon of the herb in 1 pint of water for 20–30 minutes. Never boil. Or take ½ teaspoon of the tincture. Use for short periods.

Gathering and Useful Notes
Collect the aerial portions shortly before the plant opens to full bloom, and dry in the shade. The eyewash should be made with a very weak infusion: ¼ ounce to 600 milliliters of water. As a poultice, use freshly crushed leaves compounded with oil. Do not use if pregnant.

History and Lore
The prescription for improved eyesight dates to the ancient Greeks. Through the Middle Ages it was a favorite of artists and craftspersons who suffered from eyestrain. It was also believed in medieval times to be used by witches. The name "herb of grace" came from the Roman's preoccupations with the god Mars, and it was frequently grown around his temples. In folklore it was considered a helpmate in psychic visions, and protected the medium. In a more common vein, it was believed that to sniff fresh rue would clear the thought processes and stimulate new visions about one's future.

Correspondences
Planet: Mars
Element: Fire
Gender: Male
Sign: Aries

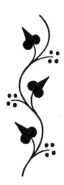

Sage

Garden sage, red sage

Sage grows up to two feet high and is often as wide. Its stem is brown with square, many-branched green shoots. The leaves are light gray-green, long, and furry. It has purple flower whorls on terminal spikes.

Part used: Leaves

Therapeutic Profile
Antispasmodic
Astringent
Emmenagogue
Tonic
Carminative
Vulnerary

Recent Research
Sage has been shown to relax blood vessels and reduce blood sugar. It exhibits antiyeast activity in vitro. Japanese scientists found a strong tranquilizing agent in Chinese sage.

Medicinal Uses; Catalysts and Combinations
Sage is excellent for improving blood circulation and the tone of the blood vessels. It has long been used to treat insomnia and night sweats. Nursing mothers have relied on it to inhibit milk flow when a baby needs to be weaned. It has often been prescribed for nervous conditions. Crushed leaves are useful for insect bites. Liquid preparations relieve throat inflammations and destroy bacteria. It is good for digestive problems and soothing for stomach cramps. Sage has a high mineral content and is useful for internal cleansing. It is an excellent menopausal herb. Complementary agents include peppermint, vervain, and motherwort.

Dosage and Administration
Steep 1 teaspoon dried leaves in ½ cup water for 20 minutes. Take 2 tablespoons at a time. Or take 20–30 drops of the tincture 3–4 times a day. Capsules are best used in formulas.

Gathering and Useful Notes
Sage can be pruned all summer and fall, and hung to dry. The fresh leaves may be bruised and used as a poultice. A throat gargle can be made by mixing 1 ounce of the dried herb with 2 ounces honey and steeping in 1 pint of hot water.

History and Lore
In folklore, it was believed that to eat sage regularly would ensure a long life. An old Arabic saying goes, "Why should a man die when there is sage in his garden?" The generic name for sage is from the Roman *salvere*, which means "to be well." Rosemary Gladstar considers sage a yang herb, and excellent for menopausal complaints. North American tribes consider it a religious herb and it is often burned in rituals. It is thought to rid a space of negative influences. It was carried to promote wisdom and attract wealth and was also sacred to the god Jupiter.

Correspondences
   Planet: Jupiter
   Element: Fire
   Gender: Male
   Sign: Sagittarius

Saint John's Wort

Amber, goatweed, klamath weed

Saint John's Wort is a shrubby perennial common to sunny fields. It has a woody, branched root that sends out numerous round stem-like runners. The leaves are oblong, linear, and dotted with tiny pinholes that are actually the oil ducts. It is crowned with star-shaped yellow flowers dotted black.

Parts used: Flowers, leaves

Therapeutic Profile

Antidepressant

Sedative

Alternative

Antioxidant

Analgesic

Antispasmodic

Vulnerary

Anti-inflammatory

Astringent

Recent Research

Recent studies show the herb is as effective in treating symptoms of depression as MAO inhibitors or Prozac. It also shows promise in its activity against the HIV virus, and as an antiviral in general.

Medicinal Uses; Catalysts and Combinations

The herb has a marked sedative effect and is also useful for pain relief. It has been used to treat neuralgia, rheumatic and arthritic pain, and nervous system complaints. Other symptoms include chronic fatigue, mental exhaustion, and menopausal mood swings. It is particularly effective for irritability and anxiety. Its calming properties are useful for insomnia and it is widely prescribed for depression in Europe. The oil extract is good for burns, wounds, or minor skin eruptions. It has been found effective for controlling viral infections and is an excellent blood purifier. It is helpful in healing bruises and varicose veins. Combine with kava-kava or skullcap.

Dosage and Administration
Steep 2 teaspoons of the dried herb in 1 cup of hot water for 10 minutes. Drink 3 cups a day. Or take 10–30 drops of the tincture. Many commercial preparations are available in powder form; follow the directions on the bottle.

Gathering and Useful Notes
Gather the herb when the flower is blooming but still budding. It should be quickly dried and stored in the shade. To make an oil for wounds, put the fresh herb in a jar with olive oil, seal, and leave in a sunny place for two to six weeks, shaking often. Strain and store. The herb should NOT be taken internally with other MAO inhibitors, alcohol, decongestants, pickled foods, or while sunbathing.

History and Lore
Saint John's Wort was used in Midsummer rituals for centuries to keep ghosts and demons away. It was smoked in fires on hilltops on Saint John's Eve (June 23) to ensure the protection of crops and cattle. The herb contains a red oil that appears to bleed when it is pinched; hence, according to the Doctrine of Signatures, it is effective for wounds, both physical and emotional. Although the herb was considered unsafe for a period of time by the FDA because of photosensitization in some people (who may develop sunburn or blisters when taking it), it has been a safe herbal healer for 2,000 years. It was named after Saint John the Baptist because the blood-red oil was associated with his beheading. Another legend was that if one slept with a piece of the herb under the pillow, the saint would appear in a dream.

Correspondences
  Planet: Sun
  Element: Fire
  Gender: Male
  Sign: Leo

Sarsaparilla

Spanish bramble, bamboo briar

The herb is a tropical vine with a long tuberous root and numerous tendrils that grow in pairs. It has evergreen alternate leaves and small greenish flowers. The plant is very thick and thorny.

Parts used: Root, bark

Therapeutic Profile
Alternative
Diaphoretic
Tonic
Anti-inflammatory
Diuretic

Recent Research
Sarsaparilla attacks bacteria in the bloodstream and is being investigated for its antibiotic properties. Chinese scientists have verified that it has strong antisyphilis activity.

Medicinal Uses; Catalysts and Combinations
Sarsaparilla is a potent hormonal herb, promoting progesterone production, and also aids in testosterone activity in both women and men (although its notoriety as a "libido" herb is probably exaggerated). Many herbals say it does not contain testosterone, but it is a precursor to it, like the wild yam. It is a strong blood purifier and is most useful in the treatment of skin diseases, especially psoriasis. It is also considered effective for clearing out environmental toxins. It has long been used in treating venereal diseases. The herb tends to promote excretion of uric acid and is a potent diuretic. It also eliminates toxins through perspiration. It has been used in the relief of arthritic complaints and congestion. Complementary agents include cleavers, licorice, and damiana.

Dosage and Administration
Put 2 teaspoons of the chopped root in a cup of water and bring to a boil; simmer 10 minutes. Drink twice a day. The pleasant-tasting tincture may be taken in water also, from 10–30 drops. Or take powdered capsules, which are best used with other hormonal herbs.

Gathering and Useful Notes
It is difficult to gather the herb because of its thick, thorny underbrush. It also has better medicinal quality if there are many roots close to the stem. It can be gathered most of the year. Root beer can be made from combining the root with sassafras, brewing yeast, and molasses.

History and Lore
Sarsaparilla was introduced into Europe in the sixteenth century from Mexico. Native Americans used it as a syrup for coughs and as a blood purifier. It was often carried by pirates as an aid for syphilis, and in the nineteenth century cowboys used it after visiting brothels. It replaced mercury for treating the disease, and caused many less-toxic side effects. In folklore, it was believed to draw prosperity if kept in the home. Because of its alleged ability to prolong life and increase virility, it was a favorite amulet of men, who carried it in a white handkerchief.

Correspondences
Planet: Jupiter
Element: Fire
Gender: Male
Sign: Sagittarius

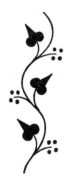

Sassafras

Cinnamon wood, ague tree

Sassafras is a tree-like shrub that grows up to eighteen feet high, with light reddish bark and many slender branches. The leaves are four to six inches long and bright green with a downy underside. The flowers are yellow-green and very fragrant.

Part used: Root bark

Therapeutic Profile

Alternative
Diaphoretic
Antiseptic
Carminative
Diuretic

Recent Research

The oil of sassafras has been determined to possess antiseptic properties in experimental studies. However, some studies show it has isolated properties that are carcinogenic in small animals.

Medicinal Uses; Catalysts and Combinations

Sassafras is most effective when used occasionally as a tea, a mouthwash, or when the oil is applied externally. It has long been considered a useful blood purifier and promotes cleansing through perspiration and urination. The oil is effective in ridding the body of lice and ringworm. It is also helpful in the relief of poison ivy and poison oak. The tea (not the oil) is useful in skin disorders such as acne and psoriasis. It has been used to reduce the pain of arthritis and gout. Its antiseptic properties make it an effective mouthwash and toothpowder. Combine with sarsaparilla and burdock for use as a tea.

Dosage and Administration
Steep 1 teaspoon of the dried bark in 1 cup of hot water. Drink 1 or 2 times a day. Or take ½ to 1 teaspoon of the tincture. Take in powder form only when in formula, not alone. Never ingest the oil.

Gathering and Useful Notes
The root bark should be gathered from live or recently felled tress, never when old. The tea can be made and used as an infusion for inflamed eyes or skin disorders. Do not take for more than one week at a time. The herb should be avoided during pregnancy.

History and Lore
Sassafras is a very aromatic herb and was often used as a recreational beverage in root beers and teas. This use was banned by the FDA after the discovery that one constituent, safrole, was carcinogenic in rats. However, when fed the whole herb, they did not develop tumors. This is a classic case wherein components isolated from the whole herb have side effects not noticed when administered holistically. Safrole has also been found in black pepper, which was not declared unsafe. But sassafras is so pleasant tasting that it would be easy to ingest large amounts, so until further tests are undertaken, prudence is still advised. The oil of sassafras is used in perfumery. The bark has been carried in the belief that it aids in healing. Columbus was said to have sensed that he was near land because he caught the scent of sassafras.

Correspondences
    Planet: Jupiter
    Element: Water
    Gender: Male
    Sign: Cancer

Saw Palmetto

Sawtooth palm, windmill palm

Saw palmetto is a dense shrub that grows close to the ground, with most of the trunk underground. It has green to white-coated leaves that appear to be saw toothed. The berries are dark purple and grow in bunches.

Part used: Berries

Therapeutic Profile
Diuretic
Yang tonic
Antiseptic
Expectorant
Nervine
Anti-inflammatory

Recent Research
There has been a number of preliminary clinical studies using the herb to treat prostate disease. Research is also focusing on its ability to regulate thyroid functioning.

Medicinal Uses; Catalysts and Combinations
Saw palmetto is a cleansing diuretic and a toning and strengthening agent, especially for the male reproductive system. It has been used to treat enlarged prostate, and assists the thyroid in regulating sexual development. It appears to prevent a buildup of excess testosterone. It is quieting to the nerves and is an effective agent in treating gastrointestinal distress. It helps rid the lungs of excess mucus, and has been used to treat chronic bronchitis. The herb is considered to be an overall tonic for the glands. It reduces pain and inflammation in urinary complaints. Complementary agents include ginger and damiana.

Dosage and Administration
Put 1 teaspoon of the dried berries in 1 cup of water; bring to a boil and simmer gently for 5 minutes. Drink 3 times a day. In tincture form, take 30–50 drops. Or take powdered capsules; follow the directions on the bottle.

Gathering and Useful Notes
The berries of saw palmetto can be gathered from late fall through January. A herbal body building and longevity formula is to combine it with the Chinese herbs tang quai root, ginseng, and ginger. Grind together and add to juice or other liquid as a tonic.

History and Lore
Saw palmetto has been an important homeopathic herb for at least 200 years. It gained notoriety as a muscle builder by early American settlers, who noticed that livestock who ate the berries developed sleek, muscular body tone. By the early part of this century, it was commonly believed to be an aphrodisiac by both sexes: men thought it increased virility, and it was used by women to increase breast size. Because it was not a plant that grew in Europe, its medicinal properties were never seriously investigated until recently. It was an old herbal remedy in both Americas, and dates back to the ancient Mayan Indians.

Correspondences
   Planet: Mars
   Element: Water
   Gender: Male
   Sign: Scorpio

Shepherd's Purse

Cocowort, Saint James' Wort, mother's heart

Shepherd's purse is common to fields and roadsides, growing up to eighteen inches high. It has an erect branching stem with many small rosette leaves and longer dentate leaves at the bottom. The flowers are small and white and the pod is heart-shaped.

Parts used: Whole herb

Therapeutic Profile
Astringent
Vulnerary
Diuretic
Hemostatic
Stimulant

Recent Research
The herbal extract has been shown to prevent ulcers in animal studies. It also inhibits the growth of bacteria in laboratory experiments.

Medicinal Uses; Catalysts and Combinations
Shepherd's purse is an excellent blood coagulant that is effective for both external and internal bleeding. It can be used for hemorrhages, endometriosis, excessive menstruation, bleeding of the lungs or colon, and postpartum bleeding. It is also a useful remedy for diarrhea. Because it helps to constrict blood vessels, it is useful in regulating blood pressure. It is a gentle diuretic and its astringent properties make it good for nosebleeds and wounds to the skin. It is also helpful in controlling bedwetting. It is best used alone or with yarrow.

Dosage and Administration

Steep 1 teaspoon of the herb, fresh or dried, in 1 cup of boiling water. Drink several cups a day to control bleeding. Up to 40 drops a day of the tincture may be taken.

Gathering and Useful Notes

Gather the herb from early spring to late October. It should not be kept longer than a year. The juice can be made by soaking the fresh herb in water for 8 hours. It can then be sipped for menstrual flooding. It should be avoided by those who have heart disease, as it stimulates clotting. Nor should it be taken by pregnant women.

History and Lore

Although the herb was known to the ancient Greeks and Romans, its antihemorrhagic properties were not widely in use until the late Middle Ages. The Pilgrims brought it to the New World, where it quickly spread as a weed. The name comes from the resemblance to the leather pouches shepherds used to carry small amounts of food. The name "mother's heart" likewise is associated with the heart-shaped pods containing the fruit. Because drugs to control bleeding were scarce during the Second World War, it was often carried by British doctors as a substitute. The Indians used it as a pot herb and the young leaves have a delicate peppery taste in salads.

Correspondences

   Planet: Saturn
   Element: Earth
   Gender: Female
   Sign: Capricorn

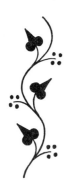

Skullcap

Dogweed, hoodwort

Skullcap is a perennial common to wet places in North America. Its yellow root produces a branching stem, one to three feet high, and ovate, serrated, very pointed leaves. It has lovely pale blue or violet flowers that are two-lipped.

Parts used: Whole herb

Therapeutic Profile

Nervine
Sedative
Analgesic
Antispasmodic
Diuretic
Tonic

Recent Research

Skullcap has been found to stabilize blood pressure and quiet tremulous pain. Some research indicates it also controls serum cholesterol.

Medicinal Uses; Catalysts and Combinations

The herb makes an excellent soothing remedy for nervous disorders, anxiety, spasms, and convulsions. It has also been widely used in pain relief, and is soothing to inflamed tissue. It is a mild sedative and is effective for headaches and insomnia. Other nervous benefits include tremors, tics, twitching, and DTs. It can be effectively used in withdrawal from alcohol and drug addiction. It may be used for menstrual pain and cramping. It increases urine flow and has been used to cure hiccups. New research indicates it may help prevent strokes. Complementary agents include hops, Saint John's Wort, and valerian.

Dosage and Administration
Steep 1 teaspoon of the dried herb in ½ pint of water for about 30 minutes. A tincture of 5–20 drops can be taken. Use as often as necessary. Powdered capsules are available, alone and in formulas; follow prescribed dose.

Gathering and Useful Notes
The whole plant can be harvested after flowering in late August or September. Although a perennial, it normally does not live more than three years. Do not use over extended periods of time, or give to children. Side effects may include gastrointestinal upset.

History and Lore
Skullcap has long been a favorite tranquilizer in the herbal kingdom among physicians. It was first thought to be a cure for rabies, hence the association with the name "dogweed." The flower resembles a cap in appearance. In folklore, it was believed that if a woman wore skullcap, she could protect her husband from having affairs. It was used in the bonding of handfastings. Those who choose to commit themselves to a life together may use it to produce an aura of peace and serenity in the home.

Correspondences
   Planet: Saturn
   Element: Water
   Gender: Female
   Sign: Cancer

Slippery Elm

Slippery elm grows up to sixty feet high and has deeply furrowed bark and dark green leaves six to seven inches long. The leaves are oval, saw-toothed, and fuzzy underneath. It has buds with tiny orange tips.

Part used: Inner bark

Therapeutic Profile
Demulcent
Astringent
Emollient
Expectorant
Vulnerary
Nutritive

Recent Research
The herb has a very high mucilage content and has repeatedly been shown to be effective for soothing mucous membranes. It is widely used in over-the-counter medications.

Medicinal Uses; Catalysts and Combinations
The herb has long been used in the treatment of irritated mucous membranes, both externally and internally. It is particularly useful for ulcers, gastritis, colitis, and other gastrointestinal problems. It is soothing to inflamed skin and all kinds of wounds. One of its oldest uses is as a remedy for coughs and sore throats. It is excellent food for the adrenals, and is a good nutrient in general. Many have called it a survival food, and eat it like gruel. Combine with comfrey as a poultice and with marshmallow as a soothing agent for the digestive tract.

Dosage and Administration
Use 1 part of the bark to 7 or 8 parts of water, bring to slow boil, and simmer for 10 minutes. It may be drunk 3 times a day. Or take 10–30 grams of the powder.

Gathering and Useful Notes
Strip the bark in the spring when the tree is at least ten years old. The inner bark is the most medicinal. To make a poultice, stir enough water into the powdered bark until a desired consistency is reached, and apply directly to wound. It can also be used on the vulva for inflamed vaginal tissues.

History and Lore
In folklore it was believed that if one burned a slippery elm branch with a piece of cord, it would curtail gossip. It seemed to be connected to speech because another legend reveals that if worn as a baby's amulet, it would make the child a great orator. It was one of the most versatile medicines for both Native Americans and early settlers. One early frontiersman was said to have boasted that one could live off of the wild herb because it contains so much nutritive value.

Correspondences
  Planet: Saturn
  Element: Air
  Gender: Female
  Sign: Libra

Spirulina and Seaweeds

Algae, seawrack, kelp

There are numerous kinds of these beautiful fronds growing in many sizes and colors, both in ocean water, and lakes and ponds throughout the world. The most common are spirulina/algae (blue-green), brown (kelp), and green (chlorophyll).

Parts used: Whole plant

Therapeutic Profile
Nutritive
Immunostimulant
Alternative
Tonic
Anti-inflammatory
Stimulant

Recent Research
AIDS virus-killing compounds have been discovered in the blue-green variety of seaweeds, and much scientific interest has focused on its role as a powerful immune builder. Many marine algae have been shown to possess antimicrobial and antitumor activity.

Medicinal Uses; Catalysts and Combinations
Spirulina is one of the most popular food supplements on the current health market. Most of the algaes are similar in action, with the exception of Irish moss (see its listing), the principal function of which lies in its mucilage content. The green and blue-green varieties are exceptionally high in mineral content and beta-carotene, which may account for their anticancer properties. Kelp (brown) is particularly rich in iodine and helpful in thyroid conditions. Seaweeds are most powerful in rebuilding a depressed immune system, correcting liver disease, blood disorders, and all degenerative diseases. They are good for digestion and athletic endurance. Other treatments include anemia, diabetes, arthritis, blood pressure, and mood swings, especially connected with

menopause or PMS. It has been found useful with some ADD (attention deficit disorders). Use with or without other supplements.

Dosage and Administration
Most algae products come in capsules, flakes, or freeze-dried crystals. Extracts are also available. Loose powders may be purchased and added to fruit drinks. Use freely.

Gathering and Useful Notes
Seaweeds are most often commercially harvested and need to be dried properly to insure nutrient protection. Use as prescribed (for flavor), but overuse is impossible. The only side effect some people report is increased energy, and the blue-green is something of a stimulant. Kelp is heart-friendly and very popular in Japan.

History and Lore
Seaweed is a very popular part of the diet in Japan, where between five and seven grams per day is consumed on average. An old belief is that if a long frond is held over the head and whirled, it will summon the winds. Travelers carried it for good luck. Spirulina is a one-celled form of algae that multiplies in fresh water. Its name is derived from the Latin word for "helix," because, as the Doctrine of Signatures reveals, its form is a spiral shape, similar to DNA. All blue-green varieties are a complete food, and much research has focused on their astonishing nutrient qualities: algae is higher in beta carotene, B12, and GLA than any other food. It has 70 percent more protein than beef. It can be stored indefinitely and is one of the most important treasures to have in the event of a major earth crisis. Research indicates that algae ponds may be a possible solution for supplying continued oxygen to the atmosphere once the earth's major forests are gone.

Correspondences
  Planet: Moon
  Element: Water
  Gender: Female
  Sign: Cancer

Stinging Nettle

Common nettle, nettles

Stinging nettle is a common perennial with a square, hairy stem, growing up to six feet tall. It has opposite, serrated, pointed leaves and greenish flower clusters. The whole herb has prickly hairs, causing irritation to the skin.

Parts used: Whole herb

Therapeutic Profile

Alternative
Antiseptic
Nutritive
Diuretic
Tonic
Galactagogue
Expectorant

Recent Research

Laboratory tests have demonstrated that the herb has anti-inflammatory properties. There is also indications that it lowers blood sugar. Clinical studies show it is effective for hay fever.

Medicinal Uses; Catalysts and Combinations

Nettle is an excellent tonic for the blood, and is useful in the treatment of anemia. It is rich in iron, potassium, and minerals, and is a plant that can be eaten like spinach. It has been used for eczema, nosebleeds, and internal bleeding. Its astringent nature makes it effective for hemorrhoids and excessive menstruation. It has long been used to promote milk flow in nursing mothers. A tincture of the herb is useful for hypothyroid conditions. It has anti-inflammatory activity for arthritic and gouty conditions. It will relieve allergic reactions and should be combined with burdock as a cleanser.

Dosage and Administration
Steep 3 tablespoons of the leaves in 1 cup of hot water for 10 minutes. Drink 2–3 times a day. Or take 10–30 drops of the tincture. Powdered capsules are available; follow directions on bottle.

Gathering and Useful Notes
Carefully gather the herb after flowers have bloomed, because the prickles do sting. When cooked or made into a tea, they disappear. A wash can be made for the hair by boiling 8 ounces of the leaves in 2 cups of water and 2 cups of vinegar for 10 minutes. The shoots are good in salads and the plant is excellent to help compost decompose.

History and Lore
In ancient times, nettles were used in weaving certain kinds of fabric. Stories were told about Roman legionnaires who used the cloth to keep warm while sleeping on the battlefield. Yellow and orange dyes were made of the roots. Although the stinging hairs inject an itching poison under the skin, Pliny and other early physicians used the juice as a cure, a sort of early homeopathy. In folklore, it was believed that to send a curse back to its maker, a poppet was stuffed with nettle and thrown over a fire. Alternately, it was used as a drawing influence: it was thought that to pour some of the juice in bathwater would arouse a lover's passion. It was also thought to attract fish.

Correspondences
   Planet: Mars
   Element: Fire
   Gender: Male
   Sign: Aries

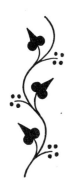

Suma

Para todo, Brazilian ginseng

Suma is a fibrous root with thick bark and lush foliage that grows in the Amazon jungles.

Parts used: Bark, root

Therapeutic Profile
Immunostimulant
Adaptogen
Demulcent
Tonic
Stimulant

Recent Research
Chemical constituents have been discovered in Suma that inhibit tumor growth. Clinical trials have also demonstrated its effectiveness in regulating blood sugar.

Medicinal Uses; Catalysts and Combinations
Suma has recently come to the attention of the Western world as another superior immune stimulant from the depths of the rainforests. It has been found to check tumor growth and be effective for chronic fatigue and Epstein-Barr. It has been successfully used in the treatment of leukemia, Hodgkin's disease, and diabetes. It has a very balancing effect on blood sugar, however, and is also good for hypoglycemia. Like ginseng, it is a good source of energy and helps protect against diseases in the manner of other herbs that are emerging as adaptogens for our modern age. Use with Siberian ginseng.

Dosage and Administration
Take 3 to 6 grams of the powdered herb with a large glass of water 2–3 times a day.

Gathering and Useful Notes
In the local areas where it grows, the roots are dug, cooked, and often eaten as a food. A tea may be made and used as a stimulant, and suma has a reputation of being an aphrodisiac.

History and Lore
Interestingly, new herbs like suma and cat's claw, which were not listed in the older herbals because previous generations knew nothing about their healing properties, are being investigated and found to have exactly the necessary constituents that many modern people need. Many who have suffered from degenerative diseases due to the hazards of modern living are finding almost miraculous relief from these new botanicals. However, suma has been used by indigenous cultures in South America for many hundreds of years. Brazilian natives refer to it as the herb that "does all things" (para todo). Major modern clinical research has been conducted by Dr. Milton Brazzach at Sao Paulo University, who tested suma on 3,000 patients with great success, especially for cancer and diabetes. His own wife was cured of breast cancer when she ate the root. It is very high in germanium and allantoin, and will continue to be in the spotlight in the years to come.

Correspondences
  Planet: Uranus
  Element: Air
  Gender: Male
  Sign: Aquarius

Tea Tree
Melaleuca

Tea tree is an aromatic tree that grows in the swampy lowlands of Australia.

Part used: Oil from the leaves

Therapeutic Profile
Astringent
Antibiotic
Antiseptic
Antifungal

Recent Research
The research on tea tree is fairly new, but it is receiving new attention for its germicidal activity due to its high percent of terpenes. Clinical studies have demonstrated its usefulness in skin infections.

Medicinal Uses; Catalysts and Combinations
The natural oil extracted from the tea tree has become a popular remedy for cuts, abrasions, insect bites, and burns. It is an excellent antiseptic and is also good for canker sores, diaper rash, eczema, and rashes. A mild mouthwash can be made and used for gingivitis. It is good for any kind of fungal infection. Natural shampoos often use it as a primary ingredient, and it has been helpful for dandruff, cradle cap, and head lice. Other applications include ringworm, poison ivy and oak, and warts. It can be used as a vaginal douche, and is soothing for sunburns. It is best used alone.

Dosage and Administration
Tea tree should not be taken internally, although commercial preparations are available as a mouthwash or toothpaste. Use as directed for external applications.

Gathering and Useful Notes
The volatile oil is extracted from the leaf and is widely available commercially. Look for salves, ointments, lotions, shampoos, hair care products, toothpastes, natural cosmetics, and vaginal douche preparations. Or you can make a douche by adding a few drops of the concentrate to a douche bag.

History and Lore
Captain Cook apparently first discovered the plant, or at least introduced it to the rest of the world, when he landed in New South Wales in 1770. The Aborigines had long been using the herb as an antiseptic. It did not gain any real recognition until the Second World War, when it was used in the machine-cutting oils in munition factories in Australia, and was discovered to reduce the number of infections from abrasions on the hands of the factory workers. Many clinical trials are now underway, testing the efficacy of the plant, which has been useful for many thousands of people as a natural skin remedy.

Correspondences
  Planet: Venus
  Element: Air
  Gender: Female
  Sign: Libra

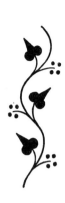

Thyme

Garden thyme, mountain thyme

Thyme is a small garden herb that has shrubby, woody stems that are slightly downy. The leaves are opposite and slender, ovate and pointed. It has delicate blue flower clusters, two-lipped.

Parts used: Whole herb

Therapeutic Profile

Carminative
Antispasmodic
Antiseptic
Expectorant
Febrifuge
Diaphoretic
Nervine

Recent Research

A constituent of thyme, thymol, has been found to relax the smooth stomach muscles. It also causes increased blood flow to the skin when applied topically.

Medicinal Uses; Catalysts and Combinations

The herb has a rich volatile oil that is excellent for poor digestion. It has been used for acute and chronic respiratory infections, and makes a good cough syrup when combined with other herbs. It can be used as an antiseptic and tonic for skin conditions. It is gentle enough to be used for diaper rash. The oil can be used in deodorants and mouthwashes, and it acts as an antispasmodic for muscle aches and pains. It is effective for migraines and may also be applied directly to the tooth for toothaches. It is soothing to nerves. Use with fenugreek for headache and ma-huang for asthma and bronchitis.

Dosage and Administration
Use a standard infusion of the tea by pouring a cup of boiling water over 2 teaspoons of the dried herb. Drink 3 times a day. Commercial oils are available; use as directed.

Gathering and Useful Notes
Collect the herb after flowering in July and August. It may be combined with honey and wild cherry and used as a syrup. It is very aromatic and makes a wonderful kitchen herb. There are at least sixty varieties of thyme. Do not use continuously.

History and Lore
In ancient times, the herb was used as a meat preservative. In the medieval period, thyme leaves were used to relieve melancholy. It was believed that if one slept on them it would lift the spirits. It was associated with courage and sprigs were offered to knights by fair maidens before battle. When its antiseptic properties were discovered, it was a well-known germ fighter and was carried by the British during World War I. It is a common ingredient in Listerine. In folklore, it was burned to attract good health and used in healing spells. Placed under a pillow, it facilitated good dreams.

Correspondences
  Planet: Venus
  Element: Earth
  Gender: Female
  Sign: Taurus

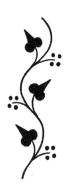

Turmeric

Curcuma

Turmeric is a perennial common to the East that grows about two feet tall and is very bushy. It has lily-like leaves, very large, and yellow flowers that are funnel-shaped. The root is orange and woody.

Part used: Root

Therapeutic Profile
Antioxidant
Anti-inflammatory
Stimulant
Cholagogue
Hemostatic
Cardiotonic
Alternative
Antiseptic

Recent Research
Much exciting research has been done the past few years with this herb, focusing principally on its cardiovascular activity and in the treatment of arthritis and gallbladder disease.

Medicinal Uses; Catalysts and Combinations
Turmeric has historically been used in the treatment of liver and gall-bladder disorders. Recent studies verify this and also show that curcumin, the yellow pigment, is useful in lowering cholesterol levels. It has strong anti-inflammatory activity and is helpful in the treatment of arthritic conditions. It stimulates the flow of bile and is useful for digestive problems. It will purify the blood and is a potent alkaline agent. Like milk thistle, it exerts a protective effect on the liver. It has been used to reduce uterine tumors, and is particularly useful for hepatitis. It is effective in the treatment of skin diseases and is a good

antiseptic for burns and wounds. Combine with milk thistle for excellent liver and gallbladder protection, and alternately with tea tree oil for wounds.

Dosage and Administration
Turmeric is best used in capsule form or applied as a poultice. Dosage is usually 3–9 grams several times a day. It may also be sprinkled on food.

Gathering and Useful Notes
The stem-like roots have been dug and ground as a condiment in Indian cultures for centuries. The curry is best mixed with coriander, saffron, mustard, and other rich spices. An infusion can be made of the powder and hot water and used as a wash for wounds.

History and Lore
Turmeric is believed to be associated with prosperity in Indian folklore. It holds a traditional place in Ayurvedic medicine. Its bright orange tubers have long been used to make dyes. Buddhist monks use it for dying their robes. The Hawaiians have used it for purification rituals. In some places, it was thought that to sprinkle the powder around the home would protect it from evil influences. The essential oil has been used to make perfume. The recent interest in turmeric has focused principally on its high content of curcumin, and extracts can be found in numerous modern immunostimulants.

Correspondences
   Planet: Mercury
   Element: Air
   Gender: Male
   Sign: Gemini

Uva Ursi

Bearberry, mountain cranberry

Uva ursi is an evergreen common to Europe and the northern U.S. It has a long fibrous root that sends out numerous stems that are four to six inches high. The leaves are paddle-shaped and the bark is red or dark brown. It has pink and white flowers that grow in clusters, and bright red berries.

Part used: Leaves

Therapeutic Profile

Antibiotic
Aromatic
Astringent
Antiseptic
Diuretic
Tonic

Recent Research

Chemical compounds in uva ursi have been shown to balance the acidity of urine. Early tests show the extracts may have antitumor properties.

Medicinal Uses; Catalysts and Combinations

Uva ursi helps reduce the accumulation of uric acid and is an excellent urinary antiseptic. It can be used for cystitis, urethritis, or more serious kidney infections. It will strengthen the liver and spleen and help control excess mucus in both the urine and bowel. Used externally, it is a good astringent for hemorrhoids. The herb is useful in balancing blood sugar and controlling diabetes. Its antibiotic properties help fight infections, including staph and E. coli. It is also useful in treating incontinence. Use with marshmallow, ginger, or juniper.

Dosage and Administration

Soak the leaves in cold water overnight; then simmer over very low heat for 10 minutes. Use 2 teaspoons in a cup of hot water. Drink 3 cups a day. Or take 10–20 drops of the tincture in water.

Gathering and Useful Notes

Uva ursi is an evergreen, so the leaves may be collected throughout the year; however, the best time is spring and summer. Do not drink more than the recommended dose, as it could cause stomach upset. It will also cause urine to turn green, which is normal. Freshly cut leaves may be applied to wounds.

History and Lore

Uva ursi has a reputation as a female herb with the associated mystique of psychic powers. It was considered sacred by the American Indians, who burned it ritually in religious ceremonies, and it was also smoked with tobacco by the Indians and early settlers. The Chinese have long considered it a kidney herb. Kubla Khan learned about it during his invasions there. The more common name, bearberry, comes from the ancient Mediterranean story that the bears were fond of the bright red berries. The association to gravel stones (or kidney stones) may have come from the rocky, gravelly places where the herb is often found growing.

Correspondences

Planet: Pluto
Element: Water
Gender: Female
Sign: Scorpio

Valerian

All-heal, cat's valerian, Saint George's herb

Common valerian grows to a height of about twenty-seven inches, while medicinal valerian can reach four or five feet. It has pinnate leaves on a tubular stem and many-colored flowers that bloom at the top of the stem in a cluster.

Part used: Root

Therapeutic Profile
Sedative
Antispasmodic
Carminative
Nervine
Stimulant
Emmenagogue

Recent Research
Chemical constituents, called valepotriates, have been identified that are the sedating properties of valerian. It has reduced hyperactivity and insomnia in controlled studies.

Medicinal Uses; Catalysts and Combinations
Valerian is a strong sedative and nervine that can also act as a stimulant in some people. (You will know if you are one of the minority of people who experience this herb having the opposite of its intended effect.) In most of the population, it is a safe, relaxing herb, useful as a tranquilizer for nerves, sedation for insomnia, and as an antispasmodic for cramps. Valerian has been used effectively for easing heart palpitations and improving circulatory problems. It will relieve gas and relax stomach muscles. It was once thought to be useful for epilepsy, although this is not one of its uses today. It may be combined with kava-kava and skullcap for anxiety or sleeplessness. Valer-

ian may promote menstruation in some women. Use with cramp bark in treating cramps.

Dosage and Administration
Pour boiling water over 1 teaspoon of fresh root. Or take 1–2 teaspoons of the tincture in a glass of water. If taken in capsules, use no more than 400 milligrams, taken once or twice daily. Less is often more effective.

Gathering and Useful Notes
Dig the roots in late fall and dry in the shade. Doses of valerian should be fresh if possible. Never boil the dried root, as poisoning may result if taken consistently this way. Valerian may be added to bath water for a good night's sleep. Do not give this herb to very young children.

History and Lore
Although valerian has a very disagreeable odor to most humans, it has long been noted that it drives cats wild with joy; hence the name cat's valerian. In German legend, the Pied Piper lured the rats out of town not only with his magical flute but also because he carried with him the hypnotic root. The Serbians called the herb *odaljan*, which means "to conquer." Perhaps this is where the name "Saint George's herb" derives. In folklore, it was a custom for women to wear it at the waistband, thus achieving the power to conquer and capture their heart's desire. It was also believed to dispel evil spirits and protect against lightening. Some Indian tribes dug the root and baked it, like carrots.

Correspondences
   Planet: Venus
   Element: Water
   Gender: Female
   Sign: Libra

Vervain

Verbena, Herb of Enchantment, Herb of the Cross

Vervain grows abundantly along roadsides in Europe and North America, reaching one to two feet on an erect stem. It has three-lobed, toothed leaves and small lavender blossoms on spikes that form at the end of the stem.

Parts used: All of the parts above ground

Therapeutic Profile
Analgesic
Nervine
Hepatic
Antispasmodic
Diaphoretic
Tonic

Recent Research
A few studies indicate that, although vervain has different chemical constituents than aspirin, it has similar analgesic effects for pain treatment.

Medicinal Uses; Catalysts and Combinations
Vervain has been used as a general tonic by many cultures and is an excellent relaxing herb. It gently soothes tension and stress and is also good for insomnia. It has long been used for colds and fevers and is very powerful in producing perspiration. Vervain clears congestion, helps wheezing, and constricts bronchial passages. It will soothe cramps and strengthen the liver. A mouthwash can be made of the tea for gum disease. Combine with peppermint for stomach problems and with white willow and boneset for fevers.

Dosage and Administration

Pour 1 cup of boiling water over 2 teaspoons of the dried herb and steep 10 minutes. Or use 1 teaspoon of the tincture 2–3 times a day.

Gathering and Useful Notes

Collect the herb before the flowers open and dry quickly. It can be made into a poultice for skin diseases and wounds. Vervain tends to depress the heart rate and should not be used by anyone with congestive heart failure.

History and Lore

The druids believed vervain had magical powers and initiates wore wreaths of the herb in rituals. The Romans made it into brooms to sweep their sacred altars, and believed it would bring peace to a troubled home. There is a legend that one of the disciples used it at the foot of Christ's cross to ease his bleeding wounds; hence the name Herb of the Cross. The Pawnee Indians used it as a visionary herb, to follow a dream quest. It was called "lustral waters" by the Welsh and the "enchanting herb" by the Celts. It was gathered and placed in moon lodges to welcome the onset of menstruation. Vervain is the herb of poets and romantics and it is often burned as an incense.

Correspondences

Planet: Venus
Element: Earth
Gender: Female
Sign: Taurus

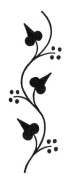

Vitex (Chasteberry)

Chasteberry, chaste tree, monk's pepper

Vitex is a bush common to northern Africa, although it will grow in the U.S. It has oblong, pointed leaves, growing in clusters of three to five at the end of the small stemlets. At the top of the stem are deep red clusters of berries.

Part used: Fruit

Therapeutic Profile

Reproductive tonic
Emmenagogue
Diaphoretic
Galactagogue
Vulnerary

Recent Research

Although there is not much available research on vitex, extracts have been shown to stimulate the female leutenizing hormone, which indicates the herb does indeed have a progesterone-like effect.

Medicinal Uses; Catalysts and Combinations

Chasteberry is a very popular herb in Europe, where it is frequently prescribed for hormonal imbalances in women. It has been used effectively for PMS and menstrual imbalances. It will reduce hot flashes and dizziness, especially when combined with other hormonal herbs. It has proven useful for cramps, fibroids and, in some cases, has even eliminated endometriosis. Vitex is valuable for emotional calmness and clarity, since it enhances progesterone production. It has been used to treat acne and other skin conditions. There is some evidence that vitex many reduce water retention and migraines. It is helpful in establishing a normal cycle after pregnancy and will stimulate milk production. Combine with black cohosh and wild yam for cramps or menopause.

Dosage and Administration
Pour 1 cup of boiling water over 1 teaspoon of the berries and steep 10 minutes. Or take 10–30 drops of the tincture 2–3 times a day. Capsules are available in female formulas; follow directions on bottle.

Gathering and Useful Notes
Pick the berries when very dark and ripe, usually late in the fall. It has a mint-like aroma. Chasteberrries can be powdered and made into tea or capped. It is a slower-acting tonic than some herbal hormones and usually requires daily use for two to three months to see improvement. Then you may never want to be without it!

History and Lore
Chasteberry, or chaste tree, originally got its name from the custom of spreading the aromatic leaves around the home or monastery to reduce sexual desire. Roman wives used it for this purpose when their husbands were off to war. It was so popular at monasteries during the medieval period that it was also named monk's pepper. They used the fruit as a spice. One ancient herbal promised that if stuffed under a pillow, it would prevent unchaste dreams. There is still a custom in parts of Italy today of spreading the flowers before the ground of novices when they enter the monastic life. In mythology, the seeds were associated with virginity and attributed to Ceres (now a known asteroid planet) as well as Hecate, since in her crone years, a woman often returns to the life of a single woman.

Correspondences
  Planet: Ceres
  Element: Water
  Gender: Female
  Sign: Virgo

White Willow

Salicin willow, witches' aspirin

Willow is a deciduous tree that grows in moist places. In some areas, it is little more than a shrub; in others, it can grow as high as seventy-five feet. It has alternate, serrated, gray leaves, silky on both sides. The flowers appear as catkins on leafy stalks.

Part used: Bark

Therapeutic Profile

Analgesic
Antiseptic
Cardiotonic
Diaphoretic
Febrifuge
Antispasmodic

Recent Research

Clinical tests show that willow bark can relieve minor aches and pains in the same way as aspirin can, but without the gastrointestinal upset.

Medicinal Uses; Catalysts and Combinations

Willow is known principally for its use as a pain reliever. It will bring down fevers in the same way as aspirin does since the same component, salicylic acid, is present in both herb and drug. Willow promotes perspiration and is effective in reducing inflammation. It has been used to treat arthritic conditions, headaches, sciatica, and neuralgic pain. Its astringent properties are good to check bleeding, both internal and external. Willow does not cause stomach bleeding like aspirin does, but it should not be taken in large doses. Combined with rosemary, it may be used as a gargle. Or combine with valerian for pain and sleeplessness.

Dosage and Administration
Boil the presoaked bark for 5 minutes and drink as needed for pain. Do not exceed 3 cups a day, and take one mouthful at a time. Or take powdered capsules, follow directions on bottle.

Gathering and Useful Notes
Harvest the bark from older branches. Soak in cold water for 2–5 hours before boiling for tea. A cold extract can be made by soaking 1 tablespoon bark in cold water for 10 minutes; strain. Use this decoction for a throat gargle and for gum inflammations. Give this herb to children in very small doses.

History and Lore
There are several varieties of willow, both white and dark. Willow is a tree common to the ancient world, as it is recorded to have grown on the banks of the Nile. It is also mentioned in the Bible, where it was associated with mourning (Psalm 137). In Britain, the trees were frequently planted in burial grounds. Willow was also associated with averting evil if one rapped on the tree ("knock on wood"). It became a sacred tree to medieval herbalists, who rediscovered its healing powers. Aspirin was originally derived from the salicin in willow before it was patented and made synthetically. The bark was prescribed for pain as far back as Dioscorides in the first century. Some Native American tribes used the trees as tepee poles.

Correspondences
   Planet: Moon
   Element: Water
   Gender: Female
   Sign: Cancer

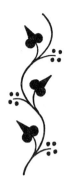

Wild Yam

Devil's bones, colic root, yuma

Wild yam is a perennial vine that grows in thickets and bushy areas. The thin reddish stems grow up to fifteen feet long and the leaves are ovate with fine hairs underneath. It has small yellow-green flowers and a capsule-shaped fruit.

Part used: Root

Therapeutic Profile

Anti-inflammatory
Antispasmodic
Nervine
Emmenagogue
Diaphoretic
Cholagogue

Recent Research

The component in yam that has been isolated and tested is called diosgenin. In experimental tests, it inhibits inflammation. Diosgenin is also widely used in hormonal preparations, since it is easily converted into progesterone.

Medicinal Uses; Catalysts and Combinations

Wild yam is becoming a favorite new herb emerging in many menopausal formulas today. It is widely used as a natural hormone, and is often compounded in pharmacies, where it must be converted in a four-step process in a laboratory. This still produces a hormone that is natural and identical to the body's own. Yam has been traditionally used to treat cramps and inflammation, as well as stomach colic and rheumatism. Use for chronic stomach problems, such as diverticulitis. It has been an effective herb for gallstones and chronic intestinal flatulence. Its antispasmodic actions are good for any kind of spasms and it is a mild relaxing herb. It has been shown to lower blood pressure in some people. Combine with black cohosh to reduce spasms and cramps, and with ginger or catmint for colic.

Dosage and Administration
Simmer 1–2 teaspoons of the dried root for 10 minutes. Drink 2–3 times daily. Or take 10–30 drops of the tincture. In powder form, take up to 6–8 capsules a day for cramps.

Gathering and Useful Notes
Wild yams are tropical and are harvested in the fall. Commercial ointments with yam may be useful to restore moisture to skin and vaginal tissues, and there are many useful preparations on the market today. See my book *Women at the Change* (Llewellyn, 1997) for more information on progesterone/yam creams.

History and Lore
Wild yam has long been considered a female tonic among indigenous peoples. The name "devil's bones" probably derives from its long twisted roots, which have a thin skeletal structure. It grows in places in the southern U.S. and was a favorite among early Southern mothers to treat colic in their babies. Mexican wild yam was used by the American Indians for hundreds of years to treat sore joints and also as a birth control measure. Japanese researchers discovered the saponins in yam in 1936 and began using it to make steroids. It was eventually synthesized and became the original contraceptive pill.

Correspondences
  Planet: Venus
  Element: Earth
  Gender: Female
  Sign: Taurus

Yarrow
Milfoil, wound medicine, ladies' mantle

Yarrow is an angular, hairy plant that grows up to two feet high with a branching stem at the top. The leaves are fine and narrow and the flowers are gray or rose with florets clustering at the top of the stem.

Parts used: All of the herb above ground

Therapeutic Profile
Diaphoretic
Astringent
Antibiotic
Alternative
Tonic
Vulnerary
Anti-inflammatory

Recent Research
Extracts of yarrow have demonstrated antibiotic effects in vitro. Animal studies also show it reduces inflammations.

Medicinal Uses; Catalysts and Combinations
Yarrow is an excellent remedy for fevers, colds, diarrhea, flu, and chills. When drunk hot, it will cause immediate perspiration and cleansing. It has long been used on wounds and will make the blood clot faster. It has also been effective in treating burns, hemorrhoids, and bruises. In some people, it will lower blood pressure. It is good for urinary infections and incontinence. It is excellent for menopausal women as a source of vitamin B1, which will nourish the nerves. It has been used as a cleansing douche as well as a mouthwash. It can be taken as a syrup for mucous membranes. It is a liver tonic and blood purifier. Combine with mint and echinacea for colds, and with hawthorn for high blood pressure.

Dosage and Administration

Pour one cup of boiling water over 1–2 teaspoons of the dried herb and steep 10 minutes. Or take 1 teaspoon of the extract 4 times a day.

Gathering and Useful Notes

Harvest the whole herb anytime when in flower during summer or fall. A strong yarrow infusion may be used as a skin and hair conditioner. For a syrup, use 2 ounces of yarrow and 1 ounce dried ginger in 4 quarts of water. Simmer down to 2 quarts of liquid and add 1½ pounds of molasses.

History and Lore

Early Native Americans called yarrow "wound medicine" because of its ability to stop bleeding. Likewise, in the Middle Ages, it was carried on the battlefield. In folklore it was thought that yarrow was the herb used to bind Achilles' heel. In fact, it was King Achilles who was credited with originally discovering the herb. It was believed that if yarrow was hung over a wedding bed it would ensure a long-lasting love. Carrying it would attract friendship. In some places, yarrow is used in place of hops to make beer.

Correspondences

Planet: Moon
Element: Water
Gender: Female
Sign: Pisces

Yellow Dock

Curled dock, garden patience

Dock is a common weed in fields throughout most of Europe and the U.S. Yellow dock has a spindle-shaped taproot that sends up a smooth stem, one to three feet high. The leaves are oblong and pointed with wavy margins. It blooms in loose whorls, usually pale green.

Part used: Root

Therapeutic Profile

Alternative
Astringent
Antibiotic
Cholagogue
Laxative
Tonic
Nutritive

Recent Research

The components isolated in yellow dock that are responsible for its strong astringent quality are the tannins. Research has also demonstrated that the herb has antibiotic properties.

Medicinal Uses; Catalysts and Combinations

Yellow dock has traditionally been used as a blood purifier and is effective in treating skin disorders such as psoriasis and eczema. It makes a good ointment for scabs, sores and boils. Dr. Christopher pointed out that it is 40 percent iron and is excellent for anemia. It is also good for the liver and lymphatic system. Use it to make a very safe and cleansing douche. It may be used for varicose veins and hemorrhoids. It nourishes the glands and the immune system. Because it stimulates bile flow, it has a natural laxative effect. Use with sarsaparilla for liver and skin and with dandelion as a general tonic.

Dosage and Administration
Put 1–2 teaspoons of the cut root in 1–2 cups of water and simmer 10 minutes. Drink 3–4 times a day. Use 10–20 drops of the tincture as a daily tonic.

Gathering and Useful Notes
Dig roots between August and October and split lengthwise before drying. Do not use the leaves; they are poisonous. A wash for the skin can be made from the tea. This is an excellent herb to use during pregnancy as a safe form of iron and to prevent infant jaundice.

History and Lore
The name "curled dock" stems from the species name of the herb, *crispus*, which refers to the leaves that appear to be crisped at the edges. There are many forms of dock, but Dr. Christopher believed yellow dock to be the most medicinal. Native American medicine men were said to keep their dock remedies closely guarded secrets. In folklore, the seeds of dock were used in money spells: it was made into an incense and burned at places of business. It was also worn by women to attract fertility. Rhubarb belongs to the same plant family as yellow dock.

Correspondences
    Planet: Jupiter
    Element: Fire
    Gender: Male
    Sign: Sagittarius

Note

The purpose of this book is to provide educational
and historical information for the general public
concerning herbal remedies that have been used for
many centuries. In offering information, the author
and publisher assume no responsibility for self-
diagnosis based on these studies or traditional
uses of herbs in the past. Although you have a
constitutional right to diagnose and prescribe
herbal therapies for yourself, it is advised
that you consult a health-care practitioner
to make the most informed decisions.

PART III

CHART I
Anti-Inflammatory Herbs

Arnica

Bilberry

Black Cohosh

Butcher's Broom

Cat's Claw

Cayenne

Chamomile

Comfrey

Echinacea

Garlic

Gentian

Ginger

Ginkgo

Grape Seed

Irish Moss

Juniper

Licorice

Ma-huang

Pine Bark

Saw Palmetto

Shepherd's Purse

Saint John's Wort

Turmeric

White Willow

Wild Yam

CHART II

Strongest Antioxidant Foods

Alfalfa

Artichoke

Beets

Broccoli

Cabbage

Carrots

Citrus Fruit

Curry

Garlic

Grapes

Greens and Algae

Nutritional Yeast

Papaya

Strawberries

Sweet Potatoes

Tomatoes

Yellow and Red Peppers

CHART III
Antioxidant Herbs

Bilberry

Blue-green Algae

Cat's Claw

Cayenne

Chaparral

Garlic

Ginkgo

Ginseng

Grape Seed

Hawthorn

Licorice

Milk Thistle

Pine Bark

Rose Hips

Rosemary

Saint John's Wort

Turmeric

CHART IV

Herbs for Digestion

Aloe

Blessed Thistle

Burdock

Cascara Sagrada

Catnip

Cayenne

Chamomile

Dandelion

English Walnut

Gentian

Ginger

Goldenseal

Hops

Horehound

Juniper

Licorice

Marshmallow

Milk Thistle

Myrrh

Oregon Grape

Peppermint

Sarsaparilla

Senna

Slippery Elm

Wood Betony

Wormwood

CHART V

Herbs that Aid in Balancing Hormones

Black Cohosh

Burdock

Damiana

Dandelion

Dong Quai

Ginseng

Licorice

Sarsaparilla

Wild Yam

Chart VI

Herbs that Protect and Strengthen the Heart

Cayenne

Dandelion

Flax

Garlic

Ginkgo

Gotu Kola

Hawthorn

Motherwort

Oatstraw

Pine Bark

Seaweeds

Siberian Ginseng

Turmeric

White Willow

Yarrow

CHART VII

Nourishing Herbs and Tonics that Rebuild General Body Systems

Alfalfa

Algae and Seaweeds

Black Cohosh

Cat's Claw

Cayenne

Cleavers

Dandelion

Echinacea

Garlic

Ginkgo

Ginseng

Goldenseal

Grape Seed

Hawthorn

Licorice

Motherwort

Parsley

Raspberry

Red Clover

Sarsaparilla

Turmeric

Wild Yam

Yarrow

Yellow Dock

CHART VIII

Blood-Cleansing and Liver-Building Herbs

Algae and Seaweeds

Bloodroot

Burdock

Cayenne

Chaparral

Cleavers

Dandelion

Echinacea

Garlic

Ginseng

Goldenseal

Irish Moss

Licorice

Milk Thistle

Oregon Grape

Pau d'Arco

Plantain

Red Clover

Sarsaparilla

Stinging Nettle

Yellow Dock

Glossary of
Herbal Actions

Adaptogens: Herbs that help the body adapt to stress. Adaptogens also normalize other adverse conditions in the body. See chapter 6 for a fuller description of this new category of herbs.

Alternatives: Herbs that tonify and help to restore proper body functioning. Also known as blood purifiers, they are most useful in improving blood composition and treating toxicity. They are therefore effective for infections, arthritis, cancer, or any toxic condition of the body. Alternatives also help the body absorb nutrients.

Analgesics: Herbs that are useful in treating pain. Analgesics may include anti-inflammatories or antispasmodics, and may be applied externally or taken internally.

Antibiotics: Herbs that arrest the growth of microorganisms. In the herbal kingdom, they include both antimicrobials, which destroy pathogenic bacteria, and also antivirals, which combat viruses. They help strengthen the immune system, but unlike antioxidants, they should not be taken over long periods of time or they may destroy the beneficial bacteria in the intestines.

Antidepressants: Herbs that help alleviate depression. Most antidepressants are best taken in herbal formulas, or combined with other forms of therapy.

Anti-emetics: Herbs that help reduce nausea and prevent vomiting.

Antifungal: An herb that prevents or destroys the growth of fungal infections.

Anti-inflammatory: An herb that aids in overcoming inflammation. It may be used externally or internally. Anti-inflammatory herbs are often also demulcents or emollients.

Antioxidants: Herbs that keep free radicals in check (see chapters 6 and 7). Antioxidants increase the uptake of tissue oxygen and help protect against degenerative diseases and infections. Herbs that are the most effective antioxidants usually have many bioflavonoid constituents.

Antiseptics: Herbs that are applied externally to prevent bacterial growth on the skin.

Antispasmodics: Herbs that relax muscle spasms. They are useful for any kind of cramps and are effective for treating pain, especially in the legs or back.

Antitumor: An herb that has shown to inhibit the growth of cancer cells in laboratory settings.

Aperients: Herbs that are mild laxatives.

Aromatics: Herbs that possess strong, pleasing odors. Some aromatics aid in digestion, or are mixed with other, more bitter herbs.

Astringents: Herbs that contract tissue and reduce discharge and irritation. Because they check bleeding and secretions, they are useful in treating skin conditions like hemorrhoids.

Bitters: Herbs that stimulate the digestion system and act as a stimulating tonic to help normalize bile secretions.

Cardiotonics, Cardiacs: Herbs that are particularly good tonics for the heart. They improve circulatory activity and may help in hypotension or hypertension.

Carminatives: Herbs that aid in relieving gas and relaxing stomach muscles. Carminatives are often spices. They also may help with griping in the bowels.

Cholagogue: An herb that stimulates secretions of bile, which is beneficial for gallbladder problems. Stimulation of bile also aids in elimination and is effective for digestive disorders.

Decongestants: Help to remove excess mucous buildup, particularly in the sinus area; also called "Anticatarrhal" in some herb books.

Demulcents: Herbs that are soothing substances with a high mucilage content. They help heal inflamed tissue and are useful when used with diuretics for protection of the urinary tract.

Diaphoretic: An herb used to induce sweating, thus aiding in eliminating toxins.

Diuretics: Herbs that increase the elimination of urine, stimulating release of toxins through the urinary system.

Emetics: Herbs that induce vomiting, especially when taken in large doses. They are useful to help rid the body of ingested poisons or excess mucus.

Emmenagogue: An herb that helps promote menstruation. They also act as general tonics for the female reproductive system. Emmenagogues should be avoided during pregnancy.

Emollients: Herbs that are applied to the skin to soften and soothe it. They are most often protective oils used to reduce inflammation.

Expectorants: Herbs that help in removing mucous congestion, especially of the lungs and throat.

Febrifuge: An herb that aids in bringing down fevers.

Galactagogue: An herb that increases milk secretion in nursing mothers.

Hemostatic: An herb that arrests hemorrhaging. Hemostatic herbs may also be astringents.

Hepatics: Herbs that help in normalizing and strengthening the liver. They also stimulate the spleen and increase bile secretions.

Immunomodulator: An herb that enhances healthy immune function by adapting to the body's needs; that is, it may either stimulate or repress immune function.

Immunostimulant: An herb that stimulates the immune system. Immunostimulants are particularly effective for conditions like infections, which require a strong immune response, rather than autoimmune disorders, which do not need extra stimulation.

Laxatives: Herbs that promote bowel evacuation. Stronger laxatives are sometimes called purgatives.

Mucilage: An herb that has gelatinous constituents. Mucilage herbs can be demulcents or emollients and have a soothing effect on mucous membranes.

Nervines: Herbs that tonify the nervous system. Some nervines have a more relaxing effect, some a slightly stimulating effect, and they should be used appropriately.

Nutritive: An herbal tonic rich in vitamins and minerals.

Pectorals: Herbs that have a general tonifying and healing action on the respiratory system.

Reproductive Tonic: Tonic especially well-suited to reproductive organs.

Rubefacient: Herbs applied to the skin causing dilation of capillaries, thus increasing circulation.

Sedatives: Herbs that quiet the nervous system. They are more powerful than nervines, and may also include antispasmodics. They can be used both for tension in muscles and for conditions like insomnia.

Stimulants: Herbs that vitalize and accelerate most body functions. Some stimulants have the clear effect of energizing the body; others improve circulation and have a general warming effect on the body.

Tonics: Herbs that promote general well-being in all body systems. Many tonics are primarily nutritive and can be taken indefinitely. Tonics may also tone specific organs and body parts, e.g., there are nerve tonics, heart tonics, stomach tonics, liver tonics, and hormonal tonics. Normally, this is a very safe category of herbs.

Vermifuge: Herbs that rid the body of parasites, e.g., that expel worms.

Vulnerary: An herb that aids in wound healing when applied externally.

Bibliography

Abrams, K. *Algae To the Rescue.* Studio City, Calif.: Logan House Publications, 1996.

Balch, J. F. & P. Balch. *Prescription for Nutritional Healing.* Greenfield, Ind.: P.A.B. Publishing, 1987.

Beyerl, P. *The Master Book of Herbalism.* Custer, Wash.: Phoenix Pub. Co., 1984.

Bloomfield, H. *Hypericum & Depression.* Los Angeles: Prelude Press, 1996.

Brown, D. *Herbal Prescriptions for Better Health.* Rocklin, Calif.: Prima Publishing, 1996.

Brown, D. *Introduction to Phytotherapy.* New Canaan, Conn.: Keats Publishing, 1995.

Bruning, N. *The Natural Health Guide to Antioxidants.* N.Y.: Bantam Books, 1994.

Buchman, D. D. *Herbal Medicine.* Avenel, N.J.: Wings Books, 1979.

Castleman, M. *The Healing Herbs.* Emmaus, Pa.: Rodale Press, 1991.

Christopher, J. R. & C. Gileadi. *Every Woman's Herbal.* Springville, Utah: Christopher Publications, 1987.

Christopher, J. R. *School of Natural Healing.* Springville, Utah: Christopher Publications, 1987.

Christopher, J. R. *Three Day Cleansing Program, Mucusless Diet and Herbal Combinations.* Springville, Utah: Christopher Publications, 1987.

Coon, N. *Using Plants for Healing.* Emmaus, Pa.: Rodale Press, 1978.

Cox, J & M. *Perennial Garden.* Emmaus, Pa.: Rodale Press, 1985.

Culpepper, N. *Complete Herbal.* London, England: Bloomsbury Books, 1992.

Cunningham, S. *Cunningham's Encyclopedia of Magical Herbs.* St. Paul, Minn.: Llewellyn Publications, 1990.

Elkins, R. *The Pocket Herbal.* Pleasant Grove, Utah: Woodland Publishing, 1997.

Gaby, A. *Preventing and Reversing Osteoporosis.* Rocklin, Calif.: Prima Publishing, 1994.

Gardner, J. *The New Healing Yourself.* Freedom, Calif.: Crossing Press, 1989.

Gladstar, R. *Herbal Healing for Women: Simple Home Remedies for Women of All Ages.* N.Y.: Simon & Schuster, 1993.

————. *Sage Healing Way Series.* Sage, P.O.B. 420, E. Barre, Vermont, 05649.

Griffin, L. D. *Herbs To the Rescue.* Provo, Utah: Bi-World Publishers, 1978.

Halpin, A., ed. *Herbs.* Emmaus, Pa.; Rodale Press.

Heinerman, J. *The Science of Herbal Medicine.* Orem, Utah: Bi-World Publishers, 1979.

Herb Research Information Papers. Published by the Herb Research Foundation, Boulder, Colo.: Herb Abstract Service.

Hobbs, C. *Foundations of Health: The Liver and Digestive Herbal.* Capitola, Calif.: Botanica Press, 1992.

————. *The Herbal Antibiotic and Other Medicinal Lichens.* Capitola, Calif.: Botanica Press, 1986.

————. *Herbal Formulas That Work.* Capitola, Calif.: Botanica Press, 1996.

Hoffman, D. *The New Holistic Herbal.* Rockport, Mass.: Element Books, 1991.

Hutchens, A. R. *A Handbook of Native American Herbs*. Boston, Mass.: Shambhala Publications, 1992.

Hylton, W. H., ed. *The Rodale Herb Book*. Emmaus, Pa.; Rodale Press, YEAR.

Jensen, B. *Foods That Heal*. Garden City Park, N.Y.: Avery Publishing Group, 1988.

———. *Herbs: Wonder Healers*. Escondido, Calif.: Bernard Jensen Enterprises, 1992.

Jacobs, B. *Growing and Using Herbs Successfully*. Pownal, Vt.: Storey Communications, 1981.

Kloss, J. *Back To Eden*. Loma Linda, Calif.: Back To Eden Books Publishing Co., 1984.

Lee, J. R. *What Your Doctor May Not Tell You About Menopause*. N.Y.: Warner Books, 1996.

Lee, L. *Radiation Protection Manual*. Sacramento, Calif.: Spilman Printing, 1990.

Ley, B. M. *Natural Healing Handbook*. Lee Fargo, North Dakota: Christopher Lawerence Communications, 1990.

Lin, D. *Free Radicals and Disease Prevention*. New Canaan, Conn.: Keats Publishing, 1993.

Lucas, R. M. *Miracle Medicine Healers*. West Nyack, N.Y.: Parker Publishing Co., 1991.

Lust, J. *The Herb Book*. N.Y.: Bantam Books, 1974.

Mills, S. Y. *The Dictionary of Modern Herbalism*. Rochester, Vt.: Healing Arts Press, 1988.

Mindell, E. *Earl Mindell's Herb Bible*. N.Y.: Simon and Schuster, 1992.

———. *Earl Mindell's Vitamin Bible*. N.Y.: Warner Communications, 1985.

Mowrey, D. *Echinacea*. New Canaan, Conn.: Keats Publishing, 1995.

———. *Herbal Tonic Therapies*. N.Y.: Wings Books, 1993.

———. *The Scientific Validation of Herbal Medicine*. New Canaan, Conn.: Keats Publishing, 1986.

Murray, M. T. *The Healing Power of Herbs*. Rocklin, Calif.: Prima Publishing, 1992.

———. *The 21st Century Herbal*. Bellevue, Wash.: Vita-Line Inc., 1990.

Null, G. *Healing Your Body Naturally.* N.Y.: Four Wall Eight Windows Pub., 1992.

Olsen, C. B. *Australian Tea Tree Oil First Aid Handbook.* Fountain Hills, Ariz.: Kali Press, 1991.

Passwater, R. *Cancer Prevention and Nutritional Therapies.* New Canaan, Conn.: Keats Publishing, 1978.

———. *The New Superantioxidant Plus.* New Canaan, Conn.: Keats Publishing, 1992.

Rector-Page, L. *Healthy Healing.* Published by the author. 1986.

———. *How To Be Your Own Herbal Pharmacist.* Published by the author. 1991.

Robbins, C. *Thorsons Introductory Guide to Herbalism.* San Francisco: Thorsons (an imprint of HarperCollins), 1993.

Rodale's Illustrated Encyclopedia of Herbs. Emmaus, Pa.; Rodale Press, 1987.

Rose, J. *Herbs and Things: Jeanne Rose's Herbal.* N.Y.: The Berkeley Publishing Group, 1972.

Schechter, S. *Fighting Radiation and Chemical Pollutants.* Encinitis, Calif.: Vitality Ink, 1988.

Tenney, D. *Ginseng.* Pleasant Grove, Utah: Woodland Publishing, 1996.

———. *Natural Health Guide.* Provo, Utah: Woodland Publishing, 1992.

Tierra, M. *The Way of Herbs.* Twin Lakes, Wis.: Lotus Press, 1980.

Tyler, V. *The Honest Herbal.* N.Y.: Pharmaceutical Products Press, 1987.

Wade, C. *How To Beat Arthritis with Immune Power Boosters.* West Nyack, N.Y.: Parker Publishing Co., 1989.

Weed, S. *Breast Cancer? Breast Health!* Woodstock, N.Y.: Ash Tree Publishers, 1996.

———. *Menopausal Years.* Woodstock, N.Y.: Ash Tree Publishers, 1992.

———. *Wise Woman Herbal: Healing Wise.* Woodstock, N.Y.: Ash Tree Publishers, 1989.

Weiner, M. and J. Weiner. *Herbs That Heal.* Mill Valley, Calif.: Quantum Books, 1994.

Weiss, G. & S. Weiss. *Growing and Using the Healing Herbs.* N.Y.: Wings Books, 1992.

Index

Water retention, 45, 180, 212, 306
Weight loss, 8, 58–60, 114
White blood cells, 94, 98, 103, 136–137, 242
White Willow, 9, 73–74, 127, 304, 308, 319, 324
Wild Yam, 176, 207, 262, 276, 306, 310–311, 319, 323, 325
Winfrey, Oprah, 19–21
Women at the Change, 5, 14, 36–37, 81, 311
Worms, 148, 172, 184, 186–187, 194, 242, 270, 331
Wounds, 99, 112, 124–125, 132–133, 135, 164, 166, 168–169, 175,
205–206, 208, 214, 217, 222, 232, 242, 257–258, 268, 274–275, 282, 286, 299, 301, 305, 312

Xenoestrogens, 13–14, 17–18

Y2K, 33
Yarrow, 68, 125–126, 148, 180, 190, 209, 253, 282, 312–313, 324–325
Yeast infections, 102, 184, 186
Yellow Dock, 114, 314–315, 325–326
Yogurt, 27

Zinc, 25, 27, 83, 85–86, 90
Zoloft, 112–113